The Complete Guide to Joseph H. Pilates' Techniques *of* Physical Conditioning

TO MY WIFE, SONJA

ORDERING

Trade bookstores in the U.S. and Canada please contact:

Publishers Group West
1700 Fourth Street, Berkeley, CA 94710
Phone: (800) 788-3123   Fax: (510) 528-3444

Hunter House books are available at bulk discounts for textbook course adoptions; to qualifying community, healthcare, and government organizations; and for special promotions and fund-raising. For details please contact:

Special Sales Department
Hunter House Inc., PO Box 2914, Alameda, CA 94501-0914
Phone: (510) 865-5282   Fax: (510) 865-4295
e-mail: ordering@hunterhouse.com

Individuals can order our books from most bookstores or by calling toll-free:

(800) 266-5592

The COMPLETE GUIDE *to*

Joseph H. Pilates' Techniques *of* Physical Conditioning

APPLYING THE PRINCIPLES OF BODY CONTROL

by Allan Menezes
founder of the Pilates Institute of Australasia

Hunter House
PUBLISHERS

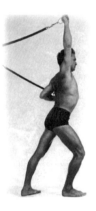

Physical fitness
is the first
prerequisite of
happiness.

J. PILATES (1880–1967)

Hunter House Inc., Publishers
P.O. Box 2914
Alameda CA 94501-0914

First published in Australia in 1998 by the Pilates Institute of Australasia Pty Ltd., P.O. Box 1046, North Sydney 2059, New South Wales, Australia. www.pilates.net.

Contrology® and Reformer® are registered trademarks licensed to the Pilates Institute of Australasia Pty Ltd. Body Control Pilates™ is a trademark of Body Control Pilates Australia Pty Ltd. Body Control Pilates Australia Pty Ltd. is not associated with any other studio or organization of the same or similar name outside Australia and New Zealand.

Library of Congress Cataloging-in-Publication Data
Menezes, Allan.
    The complete guide to Joseph H. Pilates' techniques of physical conditioning: applying the principles of body control / by Allan Menezes ; [photos, Simon Wood, Vanessa Wood, Allan Menezes]. — 1st ed.
    p. cm.
    ISBN 0-89793-285-4 (pb: alk. paper)
    ISBN 0-89793-322-2 (spiral: alk. paper)
    RA781.M4 2000
    613.7'1—dc21   00-021086

Project credits

Cover Design: Jinni Fontana
Photography: KC
Models: Simon Wood, Vanessa Wood, Allan Menezes, Jennifer Scott
Book Production: Hunter House
Copy Editor: Rosana Francescato
Proofreader: Lee Rappold
Production Director: Virginia Fontana
Acquisitions Editor: Jeanne Brondino
Associate Editor: Alexandra Mummery
Editorial Intern: Martha Benco
Publicity Director: Marisa Spatafore
Customer Service Manager: Christina Sverdrup
Order Fulfillment: Joel Irons
Publisher: Kiran S. Rana

Printed and Bound by Publishers Press, Salt Lake City, Utah
Manufactured in the United States of America

9 8 7 6 5 4 3   First Edition   01 02 03 04

CONTENTS

CHAPTER 12
Move Yourself out of Pain

ABOUT THE AUTHOR

Allan Menezes is the founder and owner of Body Control Australia and the founder of the Pilates Institute of Australasia.

While in college, Allan suffered a debilitating back injury in a rugby accident, which hospitalized him and virtually ended his athletic career. After two years of chronic lower back pain, he attended a Pilates studio in London in 1982. Six weeks of daily visits there cured his back problem. This convinced him that a huge, untapped market—people with back pain—existed for the application of this method and he changed careers to become an instructor with the Alan Herdman Studios. Allan introduced Pilates to Australia in November 1986, and he now runs three studios in Sydney as well as franchises in Sydney and Wellington, New Zealand.

Menezes has a very strong history of participation in sports such as tennis, swimming, squash, volleyball, basketball, cricket, track and field, karate, rugby union, gridiron, cross-country running, skiing, and weight training. In many of these sports he has represented his school, college, and university and set many records in the track and field. At the university level he was volleyball, basketball, and rugby captain and, of course, had his fair share of injuries.

Allan received his Pilates Teacher Trainer Certification from the former Institute for the Pilates Method in Santa Fe, New Mexico, in 1992. He is also a former member of that institute's advisory board.

In 1996 Allan founded the Pilates Institute of Australasia to ensure that quality training and consistently high standards in Pilates training were established. The institute's courses and workshops are accredited by the Australian Fitness Accreditation Council (AFAC), the Chiropractors Education Committee, and the Australian Natural Therapies Association (ANTA).

He has lectured internationally on Joseph H. Pilates' unique techniques of body control and he also conducts workshops for the general public as well as for physiotherapists, medical practitioners, and other rehabilitation specialists.

The Body Control Pilates Studios and the Pilates Institute of Australasia have been featured regularly in most of that country's major magazines and newspapers. There have also been several television and radio interviews, as well as a feature in *Entrepreneur International Magazine* (U.S.A.) in 1998.

Allan lives in Sydney with his wife, Sonja, and daughters, Jessica and Analiese.

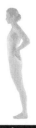

ACKNOWLEDGEMENTS

My thanks go to all my staff and franchisees (Simon and Vanessa Wood of Body Control Studios Parramatta, in Sydney, and Sefulu Calvert of Body Control Studios in Wellington, New Zealand), who have been extremely patient while this book has been in various stages of its development, for the input they have provided and for their help in the expansion of the Body Control Pilates Studios (Australasia) to the largest organization of its kind in the world. To my father for handing me that voucher that changed my life and started an industry in Australia. To my mother, who, without my knowing it at the time, gave me my best motivation. To all my clients, past and present, who have all contributed toward the refinement of the routines by allowing me over the years to test new exercises and perfect old ones. Most important, my thanks and appreciation go to my wife, Sonja, who has displayed the ultimate in patience and encouragement through many frustrating moments in this book's long journey to its conclusion. What a source of determination, perseverance, and inspiration!

I also wish to thank Daniel Mathieu for the illustrations, KC for the great photographs, and Vanessa Wood, Simon Wood, and Jennifer Scott for modeling for the photos.

FOREWORD

Finally, this book has arrived! I recommend that everyone in search of a leaner, stronger, more flexible body use this manual as the key component in achieving their goals.

The Complete Guide to Joseph H. Pilates' Techniques of Physical Conditioning contains the most comprehensive instruction on Pilates to date. The combination of precise detail and illustrations provides a clear and easy-to-understand resource for this renowned exercise program.

Those who can benefit from this book range from triathletes to ballet dancers, from new mothers to those who suffer from lower back pain.

The section on the "B-Line" I found not only interesting but also of great assistance in applying abdominal bracing in a different, effective style. It is also relevant to those wishing to study the method with a view to applying its teachings.

This book is an inspiration to those who have attempted other exercise programs and found them wanting. With this guide you will not only discover your own body but understand it and apply a process to it that delivers results.

Allan has contributed tremendously to the emergence of Pilates as its pioneer in Australia. The use of this book as an instructor's manual worldwide further consolidates his position as a foremost Pilates practitioner. Allan's willingness to share his specific insights in his teaching of Pilates is to be congratulated.

Make the most of this book—it works!

PETER GREEN, D.O.
Course Coordinator of Osteopathy
University of Western Sydney
Sydney, Australia

This book was written because of the need to have a more up-to-date version of the exercise routine developed by Joseph Pilates in the early 1920s. It is well accepted, even by Joe Pilates himself, that he was fifty years ahead of his time. Many of his advocates, who respect and honor his work, also feel that if Joe were alive today, he would have taken much of his work to the next level.

Pilates' outstanding insights into the movement of the human body came naturally to him. Many advanced instructors throughout the world, who have been followers of the method for many years, have developed those same insights. By utilizing Joe's techniques, they have developed variations that in many cases are improvements on the original. I have presented here, as much as possible, both the original versions of the method and variations that have been developed over time, including routines that cater to those with lower back pain.

This book really began when I first discovered Joseph Pilates' techniques in London in 1982. Two years previously, while in college studying for a business degree, I had injured my back in a rugby game. After several months in London, I moved on to the Alan Herdman Studios, where I learned some of the best grounding in Pilates I have ever encountered. Alan is one of the master teachers of the Method.

My rugby injury was so severe that I lay in a hospital bed for ten days and was allowed only liquids for nourishment. The diagnosis at the time was a slipped disc. X-rays showed no abnormalities, and no scans were taken. My own conclusion is that the muscles on the left of the spinal column had been so badly ruptured that any pressure on that side caused extreme pain in the lower back. For the following two years I attended almost every different practitioner I could think of in the hope of alleviating the pain.

Then in London, my father handed me an introductory voucher for this "new" method that was being taught in a small basement studio. Little did I know that the method was seventy years new! After I attended classes every day for six weeks, my back pain disappeared! Regular sessions followed for the next two to three years, and the back pain has not returned to this day. I was an instant convert. The one drawback was that my original instructors had very little anatomical or athletic knowledge. They could not explain the whys and wherefores of a movement and its application to me as an ex-athlete.

I then devised my own routines for improving my squash, volleyball, and other sports and programs for other fitness enthusiasts. These proved to be popular as more exertion was required and the routines became more of a challenge with the specific muscle usage required. (Many years later

I discovered, from a CAT scan, that I had actually herniated my disc at L4/L5! I had been living pain-free owing to the regular daily workout to which I had committed myself in my Pilates training.)

It was in 1986 that I established the first Pilates studio in the Southern Hemisphere with the Body Control Pilates Studios in Sydney. *(There is no connection with any other studio with the same, or a similar, name outside Australia and New Zealand.)* In 1994, after setting up two more studios, I established the first true franchise of a Pilates-based instruction studio, and in 1996 the Pilates Institute of Australasia was founded. This institute was created to cater to the growing demand for quality training and to provide accredited workshops and courses in Pilates.

As the demand for Pilates continues to grow, I feel this will be an invaluable text for those wishing to reduce those niggling aches and pains. It is also important for those wishing to become familiar with the basics steps in sensible body maintenance and even those embarking on a career in the growing Pilates industry. It is not only a basis for perfection in movement but also a requirement for the next step into exercising for physical rehabilitation. I hope that you will learn and benefit from the ideas contained here for a better body, a healthier mind, and limitless energy.

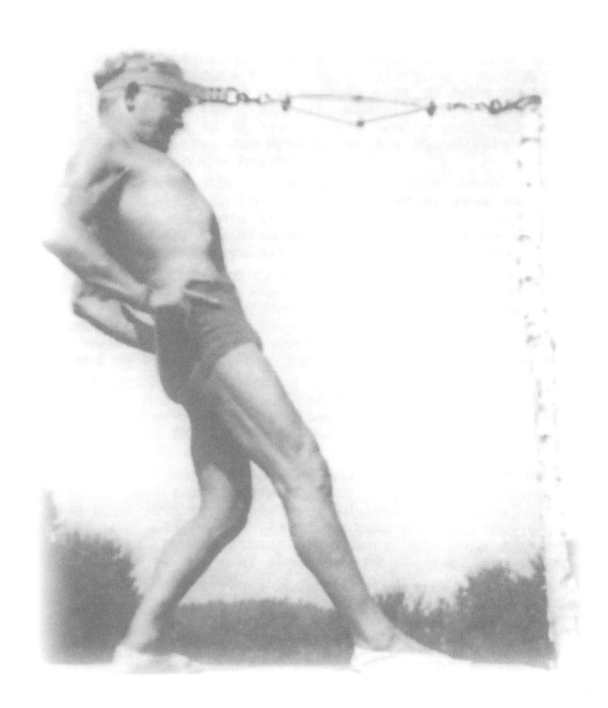

Joseph Humbertus Pilates was born in 1880 near Düsseldorf, Germany. He grew up suffering from rickets, asthma, and rheumatic fever. Like so many who have gone on to excel in the area of physical achievement and innovation, Pilates became obsessed with the frailties of the body and was determined to overcome his own afflictions. As a teenager, he became skilled in gymnastics, skiing, and skin diving. His determination and application to work his body to better health meant that, at fourteen, he was not only studying the musculature of the body but was also in good enough shape to pose for anatomical drawings. His studies also included Eastern forms of exercise. When he merged these with his Western physical studies, what has become known as the Pilates Method, or the Method, was born. Pilates named this method *Contrology®*.

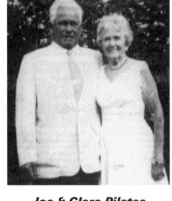

Joe & Clara Pilates

In 1912 Joe went to England, where he became a boxer, circus performer, and self-defense instructor. When World War I erupted he was incarcerated in Lancaster and on the Isle of Man, with other German nationals, as an enemy alien. During this time, many of his compatriots, following his exercise regime, emerged unscathed by an influenza epidemic that had swept the nation, killing thousands.

Those in the camp who were disabled by other wartime diseases soon discovered the benefits of having Joe in their midst. His innovative style helped him devise a forerunner of today's exercise equipment. Joe would remove the bedsprings from beneath the beds and attach them to the walls above the patients' beds, allowing them to exercise while lying down. Not only could his patients remain stable, despite whatever injuries they may have had—they were also able to mobilize themselves, strengthen their muscles, and emerge fitter and healthier than if these simple procedures had not been available to them. When World War I ended, Joe Pilates returned to Germany, where he continued to develop his work.

In 1926, when he felt his ideals did not match those of the new German army, Joe decided to emigrate to the United States. On the journey across the Atlantic, he met Clara, a nurse, who was to become his wife. "We talked so much about health and the need to keep the body healthy, we decided to open a physical fitness studio," said Clara. This was when his teachings became known to the dance world. Rudolf von Laban, the founder of Labanotation, incorporated several of Joe's principles into his teaching, as, later, did Hanya Holm, Martha Graham, George Balanchine, and other dancers.

Originally, Pilates was embraced by the dance world with great fervor. Consequently, more than 80 percent of Pilates-based teachers around the world are from a dance background. The movements, being fluid in nature and lengthening in structure, still have a balletic appearance to them.

To apply the method to a tennis player, rugby fullback, or baseball pitcher would be extremely difficult without having played that sport or having a strong knowledge of athletic movement. As dance, unlike these sports, generally places equal physical demand on both sides of the body, a dance-based instructor should ideally be trained in these other disciplines before practicing Pilates with athletes.

As the method expands to those areas outside the dance world, I have attempted to structure this book so that it can be used by anyone who wishes to learn the basic movements of the method. It is meant to be a definitive guide for those wishing to follow a sensible program that does produce results.

Joseph Pilates expressed his own definition of fitness in 1945 as "the attainment and maintenance of a uniformly developed body with a sound mind fully capable of naturally, easily and satisfactorily performing our many and varied daily tasks with spontaneous zest and pleasure."

Pilates had a firm belief that he was fifty years ahead of his time. Even today, although the original method has changed as it has spread

across the globe, the basic principles incorporated in the method still hold true. The principles have been refined over the years with more in-depth explanation of the muscles being used and the benefits of each exercise. Even the simplest of the routines gently leads you to more physical challenges, improved mental focus, and increased health benefits.

A recent report by the Surgeon General of the United States, after decades of research on the effects of physical activity and health, reported that regular physical activity provides the following benefits:

- It reduces the risk of dying prematurely.

- It reduces the risk of dying from heart disease.

- It reduces the risk of developing diabetes.

- It reduces the risk of developing high blood pressure.

- It helps reduce blood pressure in people who already have high blood pressure.

- It reduces the risk of developing colon cancer.

- It reduces feelings of depression and anxiety.

- It aids in controlling weight.

- It helps the aged become stronger and more mobile.

- It improves psychological well-being.

Gyms, with their fast-circuit classes and weight machines, tend to encourage work on the muscles groups that are already strong. Consequently, the strong muscle groups remain strong (and can get bulkier) and the weaker ones remain weak, or become marginally stronger at best.

Pilates works from within the body toward the exterior surfaces, unlike the usual gym regimen, which works from the outside toward the inside. With gym routines, once one stops, the results do not last long and the body becomes out-of-shape fairly fast. With body control exercises, results may not be immediate, but in the long run, the benefits will become obvious. When you stop practicing the method for a time, the results still stay with you. And if you restart, even after a two-year break, you will feel as if you had stopped only yesterday.

By working from the inside out, you develop a greater understanding of the body. Smaller muscle groups come into use, and you begin to discover muscles that you never knew you had—or you may realize that what you once thought was fat actually hides a muscle! Furthermore, this method develops a control that you can achieve in a range of movements—from the simplest, such as walking up a flight of stairs, to the most complex, such as lifting an awkward load from a difficult position without straining the back, shoulders, or other muscles.

The aim of the method is to produce the following:

1. Fluidity and awareness of movement.

2. Mental focus and control over these movements without the need to concentrate on them.

3. A body that "thinks" for itself.

3. A healthy body both inside and out.

CHAPTER 1

Why Our Bodies Need a Regular Fitness Program

Man should bear in mind
and ponder over the
Greek admonition—not
too much, not too little.

J. PILATES

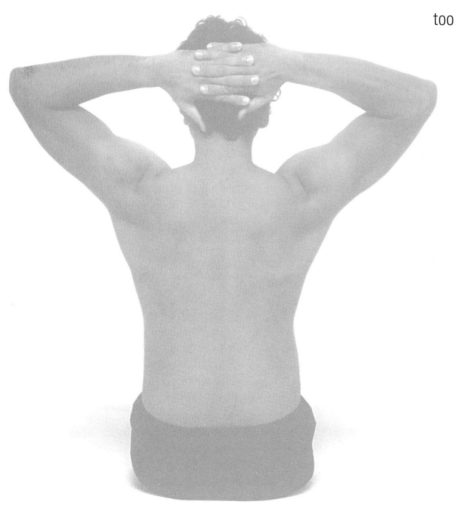

THE EFFECTS OF LIFESTYLE AND STRESS ON THE BODY

Have you ever wished for more mental and physical stamina to aid you in playing longer with the children or grandchildren, completing the daily household chores, or even playing that extra game of tennis without becoming overfatigued? Have you ever wished to have more energy at the end of each day, rather than feeling drained? Have you ever wondered why so many people accept the back pain with which they live?

Why do we act and move the way we do? Why do we sometimes feel the same aches and pains as our parents do? Why do we develop new ones that our parents did not have? Will we acquire the same maladies that afflict the elderly people we know?

To a great extent, the answer to many such questions can be found in our current lifestyle: the fast pace of modern life, our eating habits, the effects of the greenhouse gases, and so on. The continuation of this type of lifestyle can lead to mental and physical stress, thereby causing the body to break down under the pressure. This pressure then manifests itself in several forms. These can range from mild allergies to severe and chronic aches and pains, various types of injuries, or even the breakdown of our personal relationships.

These stresses can have a lasting effect on our lives. That is why we feel the urge to "get away from it all"—to escape to the mountains or the coast, to a quieter, more tranquil environment where we can "be ourselves." But at the end of the getaway we have to face it all over again the next week. How are we supposed to cope with these pressures of life? How do we control our bodies so that they do not give way on us? Ultimately, how do we live longer, happier, healthier lives?

We can usually do very little about our inherited conditions. We cannot change the color of our eyes or the tone of our skin. And other, noninherited factors affect us as well. As we develop, we begin to learn from those around us—our parents, our teachers, our peers, and others with whom we come in contact. Whether these experiences are good or bad, we tend to use them as reference points in our lives. We develop a mindset about what our abilities and capabilities are, formed in part by what we are told we can and cannot do.

As children we are influenced by the environment in which we live. We study at school and learn from our parents certain values, morals, and lifestyle patterns that become programmed into our influential behavior grid. As we see our parents', teachers', and peers' behavior, we tend to copy them and develop habitual patterns similar to theirs. As we see the behavior of our peers, we may want to go with what is "cool," such as smoking. Such choices greatly affect our future health patterns.

As schoolchildren, many of us carried a heavy bag full of school books, predominantly over one shoulder. The effect of this is the strong possibility of developing a scoliosis of the spine. Continuing to follow this pattern, as our body physically develops and grows, can lead to back pain later in life.

Various mental and emotional beliefs that we adhere to throughout our lives may then become patterns and can manifest themselves in physical ways. Perhaps because of our lack of self-esteem or our fear of adventure, our self-image becomes set. We tend to do things in certain ways and in certain patterns. We shop at the same supermarket, we go to the same holiday destinations, we walk in a fixed gait, and we move and feed our bodies in a habitual way. Many of us do make the occasional attempt to improve ourselves by going on healthy diets or making the determined commitment to go to the gym three times a week for the rest of our lives! But often, these attempts do not last long.

As we attempt to achieve more and improve ourselves, we find a constant need to refine what we are doing and the way in which we do these things. As we try to accomplish these higher goals, whether in the workplace or in our personal relationships, our physical and mental makeup bears the brunt of the enforced new routine. In order to handle difficult situations on a day-to-day basis with the changes we undertake, we require our bodies to provide us with more mental and physical support and energy. The adage of "healthy body, healthy mind" is as true today as it has ever been. Even truer still is one of Joe Pilates' favorite quotes, that of the German philosopher Schiller: "It is the mind which controls the body."

HOW WE ESTABLISH FAULTY PATTERNS OF MOVEMENT

Our workplace environment has become more sedentary, and our leisure time has followed suit. Children now spend more time in front of the television than ever before, and these habits tend to follow them into adulthood. The era of the "couch potato" has been upon us, and we have not noticed it until almost too late. In addition, the immobility that results from not using our bodies as we did before we became bipedal has not only restricted the movements in our joints but has also placed our bodies and muscles in an unbalanced configuration (Figure 1).

What this means is that we tend to favor one group of muscles more than another when we perform most of our day-to-day activities. For example, each time we throw or kick a ball, we tend to use the same arm or leg, women tend to hold a baby predominantly on the same hip, and we tend to hold a telephone to the same ear with the same hunched shoulder. These one-sided actions cause imbalances in the body. Even the way we walk, perhaps with an unnoticeable longer stride in one leg, can unbalance our musculoskeletal structures and can lead to back pain and even migraines.

These continuous, repetitive movements over a period of time become set in the memory of the muscle. These set movements, or *engrams,* as they are known, stay with us for many years. For instance, even if we have not ridden a bicycle for many years, we are still capable of doing so without falling off. These engrams have also set a neuromuscular pattern in our brain, so certain movements become habitual. These habits may not affect us adversely for years. The problems occur when we change a habit and attempt a different movement.

Our pattern of movement, then, becomes our physical "safety zone." Even if we know we move in an ungainly way (usually because it's been

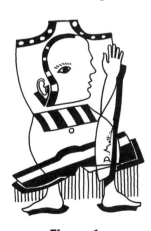

**Figure 1.
The unbalanced body**

CASE STUDY

Patient A could stand normally and outwardly appeared not to have any structural problems. However, Patient A could not touch his toes from a standing position, even after extensive stretching and exercise. The patient could stretch the hamstrings on the individual legs without problems, as these were quite flexible; the lower back was moderately tight.

A decision was made to invert the client. When relaxed in an inverted position, Patient A was found to have a marked rotation of the spine not evident in the normal standing position. After a series of appropriate exercises to counter the imbalance, Patient A was easily able to touch his toes.

pointed out to us, not because we have noticed it ourselves), we feel it is normal.

For example, walking with slight knock-knees is not a grossly distorted movement. It is, however, noticeable to others. To the person walking this way, the movement seems normal, and the gait feels just as fast and fluid in execution as anyone else's, but it is not how 90 percent of the population walks. If the gait is to be corrected, the inherent pattern of movement requires change. Even though there may be no physical discomfort, there may be reasons to change this way of walking, such as to improve speed in a 100-meter race, or to walk as a model down a catwalk.

Similar muscular pulls occur in many of our everyday movements: women who wear high heels walk with a forward tilt, which they correct unconsciously by leaning backward. The result is a forward tilt of the pelvis; the compensation of the backward lean tends to arch and tighten the lower back.

In most cases this realignment of the body's "abnormal" position to what is normal requires a reeducation of the musculature, assuming there are no structural (skeletal) problems.

In the preceding case study we see that, without our knowledge, our body will align itself according to a frame of reference. In this case, the frame of reference is a "squaring" of the torso when standing. Visual images of what is straight and correct alignment are imprinted in our subconscious from what we see around us. We then

stand accordingly, even if this is not our "natural" position (Figure 2).

Children who experience growth spurts and outgrow their peers tend to walk with stooped shoulders, so as not to bring attention to themselves when they are head and shoulders above the rest. This action tightens the pectoral group of muscles in the chest, resulting in rounded shoulders or a stooped posture. The neck may need to be lengthened to appear more upright. If the shoulders are not corrected at the same time, a greater arch than normal in the neck can occur, with its associated problems of neck pain, headaches, and even back pain. In addition, the muscles in the middle of the back, between the shoulder blades (the rhomboids), would need strengthening and the chest muscles lengthening.

In the example of the woman in high heels, various gravitational forces may tend to tighten the muscles on either side of the spine to such an extent that, even when standing on a flat surface, the woman feels discomfort in the back. This may be a result of tight calves, leading to tight quadriceps (thighs), leading to tight psoas muscles (the psoas attaches from the lower spine to the top of the thigh bone), leading to tight lower back muscles. Other factors may also influence the condition, such as lack of exercise or weak abdominals (Figure 3).

These situations tend not to be of great concern if they do not cause discomfort. However, many years of repeating the same action tends to set the muscle into what then becomes its normal pattern, and this can eventually lead to more noticeable problems.

Tightness in one group of muscles invariably indicates a weakness in another, usually opposite, group of muscles. In the high heel example, the weak area would be the abdominals. However, strengthening the abdominals is not the total solution to the condition. Stretching and lengthening the tight muscles is also of great importance in alleviating the problem. Control of these muscles on a continual basis is important. If the lower back is arched because of weak abdominals, then concentration is required to "pull" these in, even when standing at a bus stop. Reminding the muscles to do the right thing will eventually lead to a more comfortable posture. But many people find it easier to let the body think for itself than to remind it what to do for ten seconds now and then.

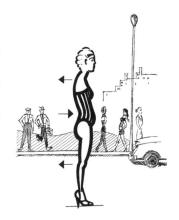

Figure 3.
In those high heels

Another, simpler, example of how we develop patterns may offer a clearer explanation: fold your arms across your chest, as you would normally do. Now stretch your hands above your head, then rest them by your side, and then fold your arms the opposite way. A little confusion occurs here. You may have to focus visually, as well as mentally, on what you are doing. Retraining your thinking to the new movement is unusual and requires effort. And the next day when you fold your arms, you will likely automatically revert to the old, set pattern. We do not want to make the extra effort. Why should we? Everything works well enough, does it not? So leave it alone!

This variation of a set pattern, however unnatural, causes confusion both physically and mentally. Its correction may take far longer than anticipated. Many people assume that when pain occurs it can be fixed immediately and permanently. In many cases, if the pain is not caused by a sporting injury or an accident, it is the result of an accumulation of incorrect muscle control over a period of time. This gradual buildup of muscle imbalance can later manifest itself in one sudden occurrence: you might be doing something as simple as turning around a little farther than usual in the car seat when you are reversing, when suddenly your back "gives way." However slight this extra, different movement is, in some cases it is capable of causing extreme pain.

The effects of chronic pain on our day-to-day

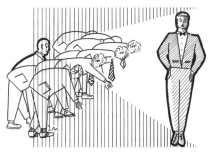

Figure 2.
"Look at the abnormal posture on that guy"

lives can be seen in those around us. We all know someone who has pain of some kind, whether it be back pain, neck and shoulder pain, or some other type. Pain can be a debilitating "dis-ease" that can be so damaging that it can practically make a person suicidal.

LOADING THE BODY AND THE STRETCH FACTOR

Prior to the aerobics craze, the introduction of Nautilus equipment, and the boom in marathon running, gyms were populated predominantly by men who wanted to show off their bulging biceps to the nearest female in sight. Women tended to gravitate toward the more "feminine" activities, such as ballet. This form of dance is challenging, but it did not entice the majority of the female population to don a leotard and tights and rush *en masse* into the dance studio, as the aerobics phenomenon was able to do.

At almost the same time, women also discovered weight training and the effects of having stronger, more toned, and well-defined bodies. Women appreciated their greater triceps definition. The sad truth, however, is that the flexibility factor was diminishing and their bodies were becoming tighter, their muscles were starting to bulge, and the feminine, lithe body was beginning to disappear.

Stretching started to become more important in the quest for a leaner body when bulky muscles lost their appeal. Furthermore, the effectiveness of stretching in reducing injuries caused by sports, and by physical activity in general, was quickly earning a positive reputation. Even major-league football teams began to employ ex–ballet dancers to show them how to stretch!

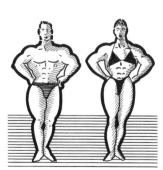

Figure 4.
"What do you think about joining a yoga class?"

Weight training, and certain sporting activities, such as tennis or golf, create unbalanced muscle structures purely because of the nature of the action that the muscle is required to undertake. For example, the playing forearm of a world-class squash player would be significantly larger than his or her non-playing arm.

In our everyday lives, the body is "loaded" not only by normal gravitational forces but also by unnatural forces. These forces include such movements as lifting shopping bags or lifting weights at the gym, the latter sometimes imposing a greater force than the counterforce required by the body to sustain a level of equilibrium—the result being muscle strain and possible injury. For

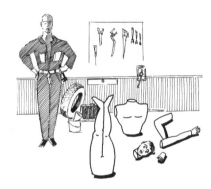

Figure 5.
Any hope in getting this body back in shape?

example, lifting or bench-pressing a weight greater than that which the body is capable of sustaining results in an extra strain that leads to torn muscles, because these muscles were commanded to exert a far greater effort than they were capable of adequately supporting.

Our joints endure tremendous forces when we run, climb, jump, bend, twist, arch, push, and pull. These joints include practically every bone in the body that comes into contact with another bone. For example, the more common joints that we think of are the elbow, shoulder, hip, knee, wrist, and ankle joints. The joints we tend to refer to less are the joints of the fingers, toes, and spine (the vertebrae).

As I have mentioned, gravity is a major stress on the body. As Isaac Newton said, "To every action, there is an equal and opposite reaction." This is true of every movement we undertake; every movement is made against the gravitational pull of the earth, to which our bodies exert a counteraction. It is when we make a movement that the body cannot react to comfortably that the weakest joint or muscle may give way, and occasionally the strongest muscles and joints may overload and strain.

Our skeletal frame is held together by muscles, tendons, and ligaments. We feel overexertion as aching muscles, perhaps after a strenuous aerobics class or a long run. Too much stress or more loading than is comfortable affects not only the muscles but also the tendons and/or ligaments. We feel strain in tendons or ligaments closer to the joint and not as much in the muscle fiber. For example, the sudden loading and twisting on a skier's knee can tear the cruciate ligaments in the back of the knee, so he feels pain in the knee joint.

The direction of the forces that are placed on the joint is also a determining factor in the resultant ache or break of the muscle or bone. In the example of the skier, he could reduce his chances of injury by maintaining flexibility in his hips, knees, and spine. Strength in his thighs, buttocks, and abdominals will give him a greater sense of balance when he's in a forward bent position.

Another important but often forgotten factor in all activities is mental alertness. It is necessary in avoiding sudden, unexpected stresses. Mental alertness can also improve physical reflexes, helping one to avoid unusual and possibly injurious situations.

Football players need extra strength to protect their joints because of the extra forces placed on the body from all directions. A football player is tackled from all directions—front, back, sides, and other angles—and by different amounts of force, depending on the weight and size and speed of the person performing the tackle.

THE IMPORTANCE OF LEVERS

If a football player were to ski and a skier were to play football, it is clear that further physical conditioning, strengthening, and a change of mental attitude would be required for each to perform the other's sport. Because the muscular and joint stresses of these activities are different, each athlete would ache after an initial training session in the other's sport.

In order to understand the concept of stresses and loads on muscle groups, we need to understand the principle of levers and how they relate to our bodies. In exercising, levers will help us understand how to reduce the strain on certain muscles by physically (and mentally) applying effort from a stronger muscle in order to protect weaker muscles and joints.

Loads or weights can create additional stresses on a joint. The heavier the weight or load, the more the muscle and surrounding structures are required to work in order to cope with the additional force (Figure A-ii). When the muscle exerts a greater effort than the additional applied force, the body can usually cope quite comfortably and bring it to equilibrium. As the externally applied force increases, so, too, does the effort required by the muscle—but only to a point. Although the externally applied force may not exceed that force exerted by the muscle, the muscle may still strain. This is dependent on the

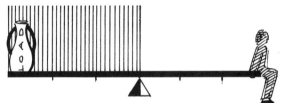

Fig A-i. Equilibrium load = effort

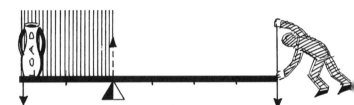

Fig A-ii. Equilibrium load = effort

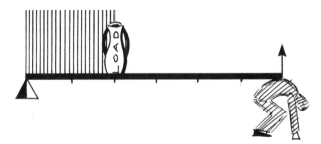

Fig B. The force applied by the load is greater than required by the effort

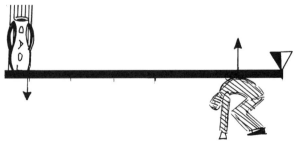

Fig C. The force of the effort has to be greater than the force of the load

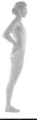

condition of the muscle and the amount of time the external force is applied. The greater the duration, the more likely the muscle will strain (Figure B).

As the load applied exceeds that point at which the counterforce of the muscle is able to contain the weight, the effort required by the muscle has to be greater than that of the load or it may tear or rupture. This may happen immediately with an extremely heavy load, particularly if the muscle is not warmed up; for example, when a person lifts a very heavy box, the back muscles may become "overloaded" and pull (Figure C). The same thing may happen if the same weight is constantly applied over a lengthy period of time and the endurance of the muscle is no longer able to contain the stress of the weight; an example of this could be holding a heavy wooden pole at arm's length for a period of time.

We can see how easy it is to strain our bodies by placing forces on them, whether internally (such as when performing uncommon movements that our bodies are not capable of achieving) or externally (such as when lifting a heavy box if our body is incapable of doing so). Our bodies require continual conditioning in order to meet the physical demands of everyday living. If we can mentally condition ourselves to perform basic physical conditioning routines that involve warming up, flexibility exercises, strength training, and cooling down as part of a regular program, we will become increasingly mentally capable of enduring the stresses of today's living. A beneficial circle of achievement!

On the other hand, if our bodies are under stress, we tend to feel pain, and this can create a circle of discomfort. When we feel pain, our body's automatic reaction is to protect the injured area. In doing so, we restrict the movement of the area for fear of doing more damage. This lack of normal mobility restricts the healing process after the acute stages of the injury. The muscle can shorten, and when we attempt a normal movement from that area of the body, without adequate conditioning and rehabilitation, we still feel pain, with the result being more protection of the area.

To overcome this detrimental cycle, it is important for us to understand how our bodies work and react to various stresses. The strengthening

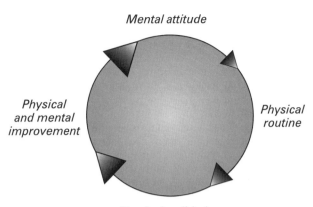

Mental attitude

Physical routine

Physical well-being

Physical and mental improvement

and stretching of our bodies, in the correct manner, is vital in breaking this cycle and certainly assists in the prevention of further injury to the same area, as well as other parts of our body.

As we become more aware of our body and how it functions, we are more likely to discover hidden quirks and peculiarities. For instance, a client once said that she never realized she had back pain until it went away!

We live with many "hidden" stresses every day. Our bodies have learned to cope with them.

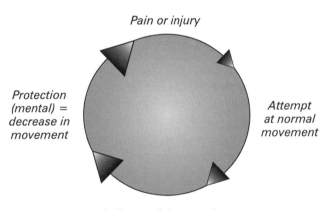

Pain or injury

Attempt at normal movement

Stiffness of the muscle or joint, lessening of blood flow

Protection (mental) = decrease in movement

However, our lives would be more fulfilled if we could control many of the subconscious movements we take for granted, movements that cause twinges (an often ignored warning of things to come?), or restrictions that prevent us doing what we once enjoyed, such as sports, or simply prevent us from feeling more agile and alert as we grow older.

Before setting out to achieve this level of well-being, we should be aware that it is a challenge.

A middle-aged woman attending a normal gym approached an instructor and mentioned that she had a "weak back." Without questioning the client about the history of her condition, or the amount of exercise or warm-up she'd done prior to her consultation with him, the instructor placed the client on a weighted back-extension machine and asked her to complete three sets of ten repetitions, in order to strengthen her back. Before completion of her first set, she complained of more severe lower back pain. With the added resistance of the weights on the upper part of the back, the effort required to extend the back became greater than the lower back muscles could sustain, which resulted in the increased pain. However, if the abdominal muscles were strong enough to support these lower back muscles, the effort required by the back muscles would be lessened.

In many cases of "weak" lower backs (usually a description of pain in the area), the opposite is the case: the lower back muscles are too tight, and the abdominal muscles are too weak. In the case in question here, the client should initially have been referred to a practitioner for evaluation before beginning any loaded back exercises.

There are no shortcuts to a better body, a new self, or a sense of achieving renewed vigor and vitality at whatever age we choose. We wonder why our bodies "fall apart" as we grow older. If we did not brush our teeth every day with a good toothbrush and paste, our teeth would eventually decay, rot, and fall out. Similarly, if we do not exercise our bodies regularly in the correct manner with the right techniques, our bodies will also decay and "fall apart."

YOU CAN DO IT!

Well, imagine an exercise routine that can give you a firmer, flatter stomach, improve your posture, provide you with more energy, and maybe even make you taller! Imagine an exercise routine that does not involve mindless jumping around to loud, thumping music in order to achieve the benefits of great muscle tone. Imagine an exercise routine that provides you with the stretching benefits of a yoga class and the strengthening of a gym routine. Imagine an exercise routine that provides you with the control, balance, and strength of a gymnast or a competitive athlete without a steamy sweat session.

Now imagine combining all of the above into *one* exercise routine. This is the routine that will change your life and your mental attitude to your own body. This is the routine that can give you increased vitality, make you feel years younger, and improve your posture while toning flabby muscles. This is a routine than can eliminate that nagging back pain and help you enjoy a better sex life!

Pilates is based on extremely sound principles described on pages 19–29. Joseph Pilates devised his unique conditioning program after looking at various forms of yoga, ballet, and martial arts, the movements of animals, and strengthening programs. He then came up with a program that was simple in its theory and effective in its execution.

However, it is important to remember that the method was devised over seventy years ago. Some Pilates traditionalists, though brilliant in the application of Pilates' approach, have been reluctant to vary the original teachings. But today we live a very different lifestyle than seventy years ago, and we have further knowledge of human anatomy and the body's ways of moving. Coupled with this new knowledge, Pilates has formed an excellent basis for the exercises in this book.

As Joe Pilates' techniques have grown, they have also evolved, and with that evolution has come a more exact, precise, and athletic approach to the method. The balletic approach to Pilates

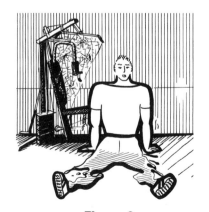

Figure 6.
Lack of exercise = weak muscles

over the last seventy years has held the method in good stead with dancers, ex-dancers, and the like. In today's environment and lifestyle, it has been important to incorporate more knowledge of the different movements required by a variety of body types. Therefore, we have not used models for the poses in this book.

The exercises described in this book have been refined and enhanced over a period of fifteen years, taking into account the athlete in every person. This does not mean that the program is for athletes alone. It has been carefully designed, in various levels, for those ranging from basic to advanced, from injured to supremely fit, of any age and of any ability. It is for the athlete in all of us.

Pilates is a safe, no-impact exercise routine that stretches and strengthens all the major mus-

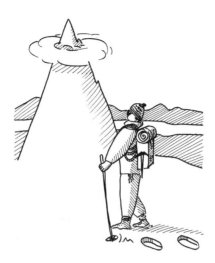

Figure 7.
It may seem daunting now, but not when you look down from the top!

cle groups in a logical sequence, without neglecting the smaller, weaker muscles. It can be customized for the individual requirements of any body.

In the following pages I have attempted to provide the most comprehensive guide to the exercises, so that many people may experience the benefits of Pilates. However, I do feel that this book is no substitute for a qualified, experienced Pilates instructor or a studio registered with the Pilates Institute of Australasia or an affiliated organization outside Australia.

As you will discover, the exercises are a challenge at the beginning, both physically and mentally. But if you persist, you will find that you can achieve fantastic results. Persistence is the key.

If you think you can do it . . . *you can!*

NOTES

CHAPTER 2

Mental Control over
Physical Movement

The science of

Contrology® disproves

that prevalent and

all-too-trite saying

"you're only as old

as you feel."

J. PILATES

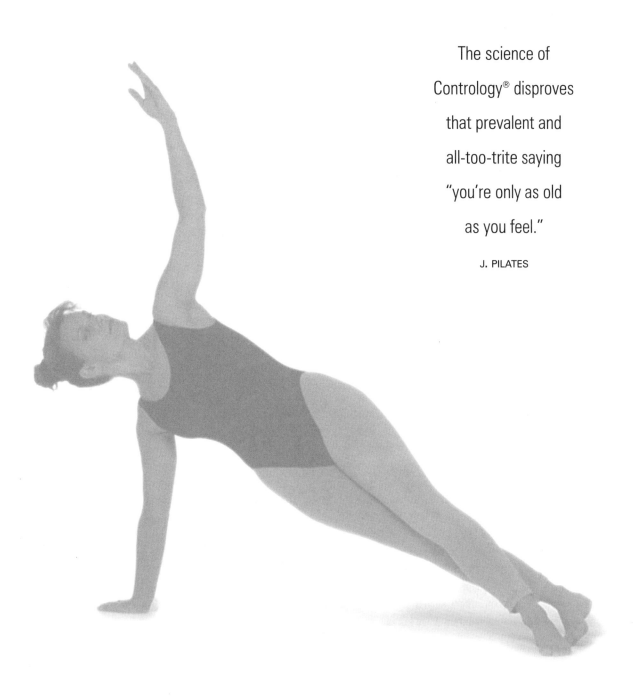

A POSITIVE MENTAL ATTITUDE TO EXERCISE

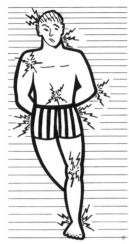

**Figure 8.
"Ouch!"**

We would all like a magic formula to ward off the occurrence or recurrence of any debilitating condition. The best formula for the reduction and avoidance of muscle pain is not magic, but it is simple: exercise, mobilize, visualize. Keeping the joints supple without putting stress on the musculoskeletal structure is as good, and as simple, a tonic as any. The secret lies not in the achievement of flexibility at any cost but in the physical control and mental understanding of the movement being performed. It has often been stated that if exercise came in a pill, it would be the most prescribed drug in the Western world.

Do keep in mind that exercising an injured part of the body, or a specific muscle, should always be done under the supervision of a qualified exercise-oriented practitioner or qualified Pilates instructor.

Before allowing our bodies to get to this late stage of deterioration, we are sent the occasional warning signals—the odd muscle cramp here, the unusual twinge or minor ache there. We tend to ignore these minor signs, thinking, "Oh! It's nothing. It will take care of itself." If only it would. We assume, even if we have been sitting down all day for years, that if we just do a quick jog around the block (without any signs of an impending heart attack), we are as fit as a fiddle and can play a three-hour game of competitive tennis the next day. We consider the jog our self-assessment fitness test—and we passed! Our mental power, in its limited capacity, has told us that, without any serious aftereffects, we have the athletic capability of a teenager.

With minimal warming up and less-than-adequate stretching, we then proceed to push our bodies to the limits of the physical challenges of the day. We would be surprised if we were not aching the following day. "This must be good," we say to ourselves, "I have worked my muscles really well." And then, we remain inactive until the same time the following week.

The infrequency with which we tend to our bodies is scandalous. We care for our cars better than we care for the far more complex "machines" of our bodies, with so many thousands more delicate parts.

Anything more serious than the occasional ache or pain and we shuffle off to the doctor, or some health practitioner, who prescribes a concoction of tablets whose names we cannot pronounce, or treats the affected area, which has been aching for days, in under an hour. We feel better and assume the problem is fixed for good.

Unfortunately, for most of us, this is our body's first warning of the beginning of the decay process. This "decay" does not necessarily take place throughout the entire body at the same time. It could be a knee problem here, a neck problem there. We may not feel it until we slow down and stop the regular physical activity we had done for years before.

Little wonder that we were once able to get through high-impact aerobic sessions with such ease, yet some years after we have stopped, without much strenuous activity, we find that we are suddenly starting to fall apart.

The reason for this is simple. The wear and tear that the body and its joints have been subject to for many years is just beginning to show through. Combine these ingredients with the lack of safe, regular stretching and conditioning programs, and we have a recipe for immobility, discomfort, and, too frequently, pain.

In years gone by, we were capable of pushing our bodies without too much warming up. And

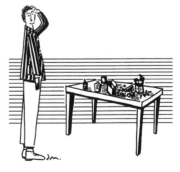

**Figure 9.
Jim the Junkie—deciding which tablet
keeps him the fittest!**

our bodies were able to withstand these pressures. The young muscles can easily cope with spontaneous strenuous activity. The energy levels of our adolescent years seem to remain in our memory banks years after they have actually diminished.

Unfortunately, we still think we have this endless source of youthful vigor without having to work to maintain it or "keep those batteries charged." On a pleasant, sunny afternoon with friends we still feel capable of overreaching for that elusive kick or hit of the soccer ball, tennis ball, or volleyball. Ouch! Too late. The damage is done. We feel a sharp pain in the back, hamstring, or shoulder, yet we continue to play, because we feel we are fit (or we wish to appear so to those around us). The pain is bearable. We retire to bed and trust that a good night's rest will see us well in the morning. Morning arrives—and we cannot move!

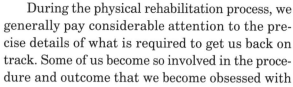

**Figure 10.
This body is as
young as ever**

These signs of aging do not affect only us mere mortals. We see it in all professions. Even ballet dancers, who are the epitome of flexibility and fitness to most of us, acquire creaky hip, knee, and ankle joints later in life. No one is able to escape the onset of old age. However, there are solutions to cope with this onset of physical senility, so that we can enjoy life in a more pain-free and fulfilling manner.

THE MENTAL FACTOR

*By reawakening thousands and thousands
of otherwise ordinary dormant muscle cells,
Contrology® correspondingly reawakens
thousands and thousands of dormant brain
cells, thus activating new areas and stimulating
further the functioning of the mind.*

J. PILATES

Our general mental attitude to our bodies is one of invincibility. When our bodies fail us, we are somewhat surprised. An injury that lays us low, or even hospitalizes us, can be emotionally devastating. In many instances, the grieving we go through after an injury has immobilized us, if we were physically active, can parallel that of losing a loved one.

During the physical rehabilitation process, we generally pay considerable attention to the precise details of what is required to get us back on track. Some of us become so involved in the procedure and outcome that we become obsessed with how it all works. We become more knowledgeable about muscles, injury, and the curing of our particular complaint. We become so expert in the field that we even go as far as to advise others with similar conditions!

We are more capable of achieving results after injury because we are determined to overcome this affliction. We become mentally focused on our goal. But this mental focus and determination can also be used when we are not injured. It can be used to prevent injuries from happening in the first place, as well as helping to speed up rehabilitation after an injury. It can be used to gain greater control over weak muscle groups. It can be used to improve our performance in whatever sport or movement we desire.

Developing a "Thinking Body"

*Contrology® begins with
mind control over muscles.*

J. PILATES

Concentrating on the precision of what we are physically doing will also make us mentally alert. This takes practice and repetition. To be in control of our bodies involves understanding what we are currently capable of achieving, and how we can safely extend these limits. We need to achieve a "thinking body," one that is eventually able to control movements, however demanding, with precision, control, and fluidity without our having to think consciously about the demands of the movement. This requires mental focus.

To develop the thinking body, we need to understand the body itself: the major muscle groups and their functions, and how these affect physical outcomes. To that end, I have provided the following list of terms. The purpose here is to give you a broad understanding of these areas without becoming too clinical in the approach. Many of you who have suffered injuries will already be familiar with these terms.

MOVEMENT TERMS

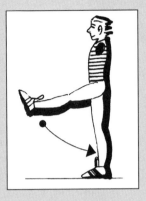

Extension means lengthening out or straightening.

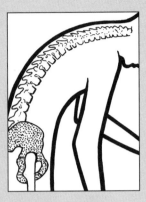

Flexion means folding or bending. Flexors of the toes curl the toes.

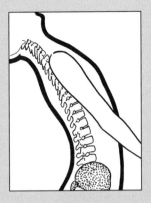

Hyperextension means extending more than 180 degrees.

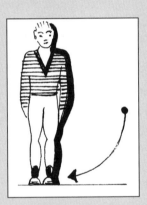

Adduction means movement that draws inward (toward the midline of the body).

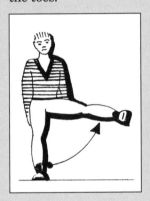

Abduction means movement that draws away (from the mid-line of the body).

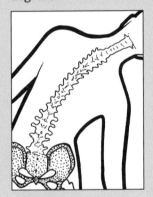

Lateral flexion is a side bend of the body. Adductors and abductors oppose one another.

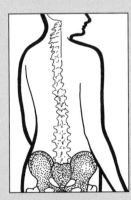

Rotation means movement around the central axis of a lever.

ANATOMICAL TERMS

Tendon: elastic connective tissue that connects muscle to bone.

Ligament: nonelastic connective tissue that connects bone to bone.

Lordosis: the hyperextension of the normal curve in the lumbar or cervical spine.

Kyphosis: the forward flexion of the normal thoracic curve of the spine.

Scoliosis: lateral curvature of the spine.

Supine: on the back.

Prone: on the stomach.

Range of motion/movement (ROM): the degree to which a limb may comfortably move around a joint without affecting other parts of the body.

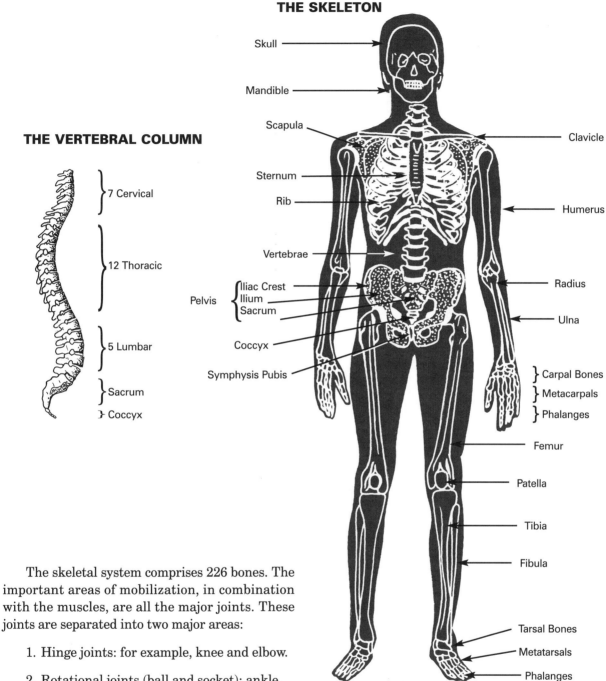

THE SKELETON

- Skull
- Mandible
- Scapula
- Clavicle
- Sternum
- Rib
- Humerus
- Vertebrae
- Pelvis
  - Iliac Crest
  - Ilium
  - Sacrum
- Radius
- Ulna
- Coccyx
- Symphysis Pubis
- Carpal Bones
- Metacarpals
- Phalanges
- Femur
- Patella
- Tibia
- Fibula
- Tarsal Bones
- Metatarsals
- Phalanges

THE VERTEBRAL COLUMN

- 7 Cervical
- 12 Thoracic
- 5 Lumbar
- Sacrum
- Coccyx

The skeletal system comprises 226 bones. The important areas of mobilization, in combination with the muscles, are all the major joints. These joints are separated into two major areas:

1. Hinge joints: for example, knee and elbow.

2. Rotational joints (ball and socket): ankle, hip, shoulder, wrist.

The entire skeleton is held together by muscles, tendons and ligaments, and connective tissue. Without this the skeleton, we would simply fall to the floor because of the gravitational pull of the earth. The skeleton has several important functions:

1. It acts as a framework to support the softer parts of the body.

2. It protects the more delicate areas of our body, such as the brain, heart, lungs, and spinal cord.

3. It helps to produce blood cells in the bones, which contain red marrow.

4. Together with the contraction of the muscles, it allows us to move.

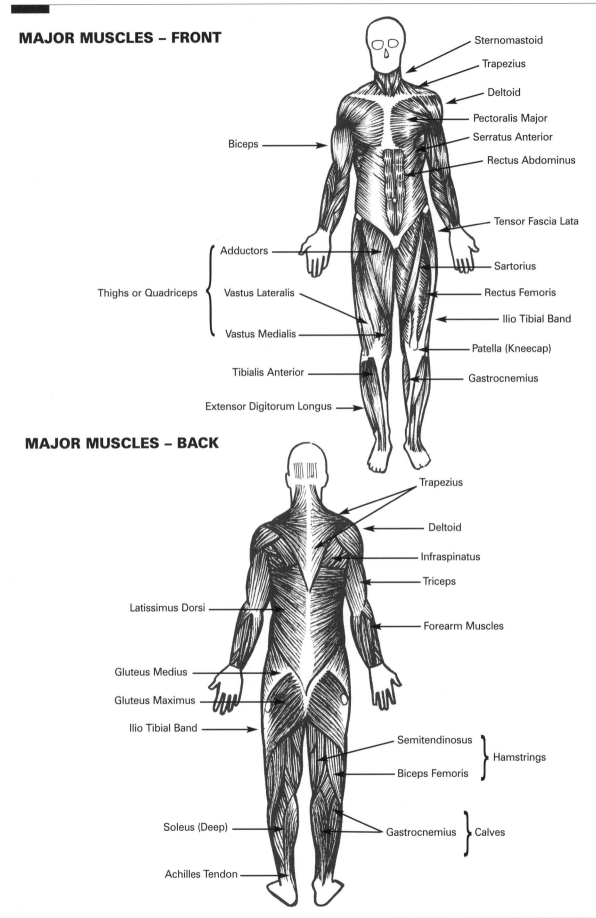

MAJOR MUSCLES – FRONT

- Sternomastoid
- Trapezius
- Deltoid
- Pectoralis Major
- Serratus Anterior
- Rectus Abdominus
- Biceps
- Tensor Fascia Lata
- Adductors
- Sartorius
- Thighs or Quadriceps
- Vastus Lateralis
- Rectus Femoris
- Ilio Tibial Band
- Vastus Medialis
- Patella (Kneecap)
- Tibialis Anterior
- Gastrocnemius
- Extensor Digitorum Longus

MAJOR MUSCLES – BACK

- Trapezius
- Deltoid
- Infraspinatus
- Triceps
- Latissimus Dorsi
- Forearm Muscles
- Gluteus Medius
- Gluteus Maximus
- Ilio Tibial Band
- Semitendinosus
- Hamstrings
- Biceps Femoris
- Soleus (Deep)
- Gastrocnemius
- Calves
- Achilles Tendon

THE EIGHT PRINCIPLES OF THE METHOD

To understand Pilates' method, we first need to understand the principles behind the technique and why they are so essential. Not understanding the essentials is akin to attempting to drive a car without the engine; you may cruise along the flats, but it becomes extremely hard work when it comes to the hills!

The manner in which the exercises are performed is of far greater importance than the number of repetitions or the amount of exertion applied to the movements. Quality is superior to quantity. In fact, to master a simple movement is sometimes more difficult than to force the body to perform tasks beyond its normal capabilities. By combining application and dedication to the basic principles, you can more easily achieve the desired results. Attaining the body that one desires is not as scientific or mind-bending as many people think.

The eight principles are:

1. Concentration

2. Centering

3. Breathing

4. Control (including strength)

5. Precision

6. Flowing Movement

7. Isolation (including flexibility)

8. Routine

These eight principles may, at first, appear simple and logical in their individual parts. But it can be challenging to remember all of them at the same time when performing even a simple exercise. When you first begin the program, focusing on even two of them may require some effort. Slowly, as you are able to master one principle at a time with some of the more basic exercises, you will discover the enormous effect that even a slight variation of the movement can have on the effort required to perform that movement.

It is the mind's subconscious control over habitual movements that needs to be altered to progress above and beyond our standard capabilities.

As the exercises are more readily mastered, we are capable of achieving more than we have previously accomplished. This may take some time. As we follow the exercises that we find are easily performed, more challenging versions are suggested. As we perform the routines on a regular basis, we discover that at the end of a session our energy levels increase as we achieve more. The days do not seem as long, and we look forward to physical and mental challenges without regarding them as insurmountable problems. We perceive them as challenges with a natural solution. We sleep better, we awake more refreshed, our physical and mental reflexes are more highly tuned.

Frederich von Schiller, an eighteenth-century German philosopher, once said, "It is the mind itself which builds the body." With Joseph Pilates' techniques, we are not only exercising our body but also simultaneously exercising our mind.

1. CONCENTRATION

Concentrate on the correct movements each time you exercise, lest you do them improperly and thus lose all the vital benefits of their value.
J. PILATES

Concentration with regard to body movement is required at all times. To focus on muscles as they move is not an easy task to master initially, as the body does not easily follow what the mind wants it to do. If the muscles in question have not been often used before, the initial movement is awkward and jerky. Once we achieve continual mental attention and focus, we see that what once appeared to be simple movements are actually quite complex.

The first step of the process is the realization that the position and the movement of every part of the body is of great importance, and that all the movements and positions are interconnected. When we walk or run, or when we reach for a cup of coffee, the positioning of the foot or arm is both influenced and affected by the correct alignment of the body.

To concentrate on the entire body at the same time as it performs complex movements is a formidable challenge and takes time. It is a skill you will acquire as the method becomes more familiar. By focusing your attention on specific muscles, you

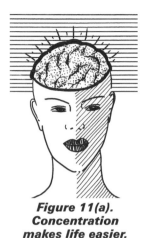

Figure 11(a). Concentration makes life easier.

train the mental process to become more tuned-in. As these movements begin to achieve a level of precision, the results are more noticeable.

Concentration is required when following each of the other seven principles. Each principle becomes clearer and more focused with the improved concentration that is required. In addition, your thinking becomes clearer, and you become more focused on other issues when outside the studio or exercise environment.

The benefits of concentration are somewhat obvious: clarity of thought; better mental focus, leading to increased mental energy; increased ability to handle difficult situations more calmly and positively; fresh approaches to new and unusual conditions; the list goes on…. You will discover, even at the start of the routines, that in order to accomplish even the most simple of exercises our mind needs to focus on small movements.

We need to alter the physical (restrictive) patterns that have become embodied in our subconscious. In some cases, this can be quite demanding, requiring effort and determination to correct imbalances that have been present for months, or even years. This focus while the body is in motion requires just that much more mental energy. Over time, like the benefits of the exercises themselves, this meditative effect slowly seeps its way into the subconscious, and the entire body and mind become more energized after the exercise routine.

As we correctly perform the movements, we find that we are unable to think of other things that have happened during the day. We eliminate problems from our mind. We truly give this time to ourselves.

2. CENTERING

The abdominal area is often described as the second spine. It is the powerhouse of the anatomy. The center is described as the area between the

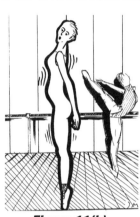

Figure 11(b). Dancer—potbelly

ribs and the hips at both anterior (front) and posterior (back) parts of the torso. A strong center is also important to maintaining good control and balance in the body as a whole. It provides assistance for movements both slow and fast, such as balancing on a beach ball or sprinting one hundred meters.

Imagine a ballet dancer standing on one leg on *pointe* (on the toes), with the other leg pointed to the ceiling and her arms above her head—and loose abdominals (or worse still, a potbelly!). She would fall over instantly.

The center is the pivotal point of the body. All strength movements emanate from this area. In karate, the *Ki* (life force, energy) comes from the solar plexus. The efforts of movement, force, balance, and strength come from the center.

Abdominal control is different from abdominal strength. However, the former does rely on the latter. It is preferable to have control. In many

CASE STUDY

Tennis players do most of their abdominal strength work by performing crunches with the knees bent. When they stand up, their abdominal muscles are more lengthened and have less strength than they did in the position in which they were worked. As a result, when players serve, the abdominal muscles are at full stretch. There is no strength from their center to perform this movement efficiently and effectively. The majority of the force for the serve then comes from the shoulder and arm. If the abdominals were strengthened when at full stretch, the center could be brought into play and the serve would become more effective. This also applies to the majority of sports.

workout routines, most of the abdominal strength is achieved by performing crunches, sit-ups, or some manner of forward contraction or flexion of the body. This limits the control of the abdominals and most of their strength to that position where the abdominal contraction takes place: a forward curved position of the torso. Abdominal strength provides support, while abdominal control provides fluidity of movement from the center.

The "B-Line"

Using the "B-Line" is an age-old Pilates approach to abdominal control; the emphasis here is on the exactness of the movement and how best to engage the lower abdominals. The B-Line, together with correct foot placement, is the foundation of good posture. (See "The Tripod Position," in Chapter 3.)

Do the following:

1. Stand upright, with your feet hip-distance apart.

2. Draw the abdominals as close to the spine as possible and breathe normally.

What do you feel?
You may notice several things:

1. The area drawing to the spine is generally the navel, or middle and upper abdominals, with some lower abdominal connection.

2. The pelvis may be tucked to provide a feeling of flattening the back (this especially happens when lying on the floor or standing against a wall).

3. The knees may bend slightly or the shoulders round. The ribs slightly drop to the hips.

4. The buttocks may be clenched.

5. Breathing may be somewhat restricted, with a feeling of forcing the breath into the lungs.

6. There is generally little or no feeling of abdominal contraction in the area below the navel.

Now, abolish all thoughts of drawing the navel to the spine!

Stand as before and relax. Now, do the following, without clenching the buttocks, tucking the pelvis, or dropping the shoulders:

1. With your finger, trace a straight line from the top of one hipbone to the other (see diagram). You may notice that the line is in front of the hipbones (Figure12(i)).

2. Go to the center of this line (2 to 3 inches below the belly button) and draw the stomach in behind the line of the hips (hence, the B-Line) and away from your finger.

When was the last time you felt these lower abdominal muscles working?

This is the B-Line. *Maintain this for the rest of your life!* We shall be using this term throughout the book. Initially, you may feel some mild discomfort in the lower back. This will diminish as your body becomes used to this new positioning.

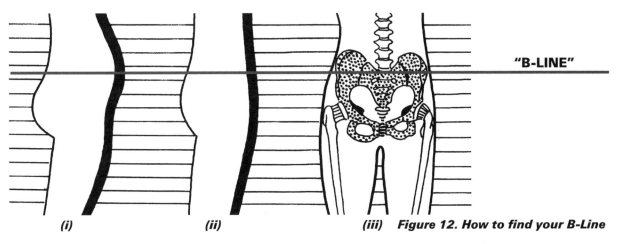

"B-LINE"

(i)   *(ii)*   *(iii)*   **Figure 12. How to find your B-Line**

You may notice that you may be standing a little more upright. Your breathing may still feel restricted. Be sure to breathe as described in the section below on breathing.

An Example of the B-Line in Action

Stand up out of a chair. You may notice that your upper body leaned forward over the knees first, before coming to the standing position. Take a seat again, and now get your body into a B-Line before you rise up out of the chair. You may notice that you stood up without leaning forward so far, and your back may have felt more supported.

The Perfect Abdominal Curl

When working the abdominal muscles to gain strength in exercises involving a forward contraction, such as roll-ups, sit-ups, or maintaining a contracted position, there is a definite sequence of movements to follow.

The first movement, even before the head is raised off the floor, is the B-Line. This also has a significant benefit in that it creates pressure against the psoas (see "Muscle Imbalances," pp. 34–36) and reduces its pull, thereby reducing stiffness, or an arch, in the lower back. The tailbone is not tilted to the ceiling. This gives a false impression of keeping the back flat.

1. Keep the knees bent at a right angle at the knee joint, or farther, as long as the lower back remains flat, without tucking the pelvis or pressing the feet into the floor. Keep the feet flexed and the eyes above the knees.

2. Draw the rib cage toward the hips and scoop the abdominals. This action brings the head and shoulders forward without the usual strain in the neck. When performing the curl, draw the ribs toward the hips as close as possible in a horizontal plane, breathing out deeply. When releasing, relax only 10 percent of the contraction before repeating the movement. The shoulder blades should never rest on the floor at any time until all repetitions are complete. If they do, they release the control of the abdominals and they almost rest!

Nine times out of ten, people perform crunches by first lifting the head and shoulders forward. If you allow this reflex action to dominate, the abdominals will usually bulge out, and

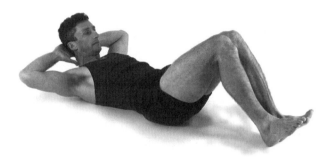

after a while, the neck and shoulders start to strain. Many people have said that they perform hundreds of crunches but still have back pain! As long as the ribs are drawn to the hips in the same plane, with the abdominals scooped (try to imagine copying a greyhound's stomach!), the abdominals will perform their function correctly. But when the ribs lift above the level of the hips, then the hip flexors engage and the back stiffens to perform a lift. The purpose of the curl is then defeated, and the abdominals do not perform to 100 percent capacity.

3. BREATHING

To breathe correctly you must completely exhale and inhale, always trying very hard to "squeeze" every atom of impure air from your lungs in much the same manner that you would wring every drop of water from a wet cloth.

J. PILATES

Breathing is the most important physical principle to refine before attempting an exercise or movement. Breathing has three major functions:

1. To carry nutrients to all parts of the body, thereby charging the whole body with more energy.

2. To carry away wastes for elimination from the body.

3. To increase stamina.

Wastes can produce restrictions within the body's system. These can be various, such as tightness and restricted movement in joints,

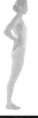

tiredness, headaches, and pain. This is not to say that breathing on its own can cure these conditions—it cannot. But, combined with the other principles, it can certainly lead to greater well-being. Drinking the required quantity of water (eight glasses per day) to assist in waste elimination also helps greatly in achieving this goal. It has also been suggested that adequate water consumption can improve flexibility of the muscles.

As we have all seen in gym and other (weight) training situations, many people hold their breath at the most crucial part of the exercise, when it could be most beneficial. You have probably been guilty of this yourself, in the past, without realizing it. When we do this, we put our bodies under an enormous amount of physical tension, especially in the upper thoracic and cervical area.

When we hold the breath while exercising, we create a situation similar to that of pressure building up inside a pressure cooker. As a result, we waste energy and effort on a part, or parts, of the body where they are not required. The outcome is less-than-efficient utilization of the muscles being worked as the subconscious mental concentration becomes more focused on the stress the body is undergoing.

Try this simple exercise. Breathe in as you raise your arms above your head. Press your arms to your sides, as if through a vat of molasses. As you lower your arms, hold your breath for as long as you can. Can you feel the tension in your neck and shoulders? Now repeat the same exercise, but as you lower your arms, gradually let the breath out in a long sigh. Can you feel how much more relaxing this is?

Correct breathing should be performed with the following in mind:

1. Keep the neck and shoulders relaxed; hunching causes neck tension.

2. Allow the breath to flow: don't hold your breath at any point.

3. Breathe in through the nose (into the chest) for a five-second count, without allowing the shoulders to lift at all (try this in front of a mirror and keep an eye on your shoulders).

4. Without stopping, breathe out of the mouth with a sigh for a five-second count (drop the jaw and do not purse the lips into any shape). Breathing out through your teeth, with your lips pursed, with your jaw clenched, or with your cheeks puffed does not allow all the air to be expelled from the bottom of the lungs. It also tenses the neck, jaw, and face. This unnecessary contortion of the breathing leads to waste of energy in an area that does not need to be worked. This energy can be better utilized in the performance of the exercise itself.

5. If you find it difficult to breathe into the chest, breathe "into your back" or shoulder blades as if there were a deflated balloon in this area. Many people forget that there is a whole section of space in the back of our chest cavity for extra breath intake!

Try this method of breathing, along with the B-Line, in the following exercise. Notice how much less restricted your breath feels, and how much deeper a breath you can take. This is important in increasing lung capacity and improving stamina.

Breathing Exercise

Sit down with your legs comfortably crossed in front of you. Sit as upright as possible, as if your lower back were being supported by a wall, with no gaps between your tailbone and the wall. Do not lean into the wall. Place your hands snugly just below your navel. Without hunching the shoulders, take a five-second breath in through the nose and let out a five-second sigh from the mouth. You may notice that on the breath in you felt the stomach move outward, and on the breath out it went down. (If five seconds is too long for the breath in, attempt four seconds.)

Now repeat the same exercise, except before you breathe in, press your hands very firmly on the B-Line below the navel, against your lower abdominals and towards your spine, and keep them there. Now breathe into your chest. You will find that this is quite difficult to achieve without the hands moving at all. You may also find that the breath into the chest is quite restricted and that there is a slight sensation of "choking" the breath into your chest.

These things happen because as we reduce

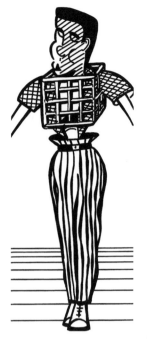

**Figure 13.
Restricted
breathing**

our exercise levels, our breathing capacity reduces. If we return to our usual level of exercise after a long break we find that, in a short space of time, we are gasping for breath. As we tend to do less abdominal work, we tend to breathe more into the stomach and thus loosen the abdominal muscles. As this happens, the usually pliable, intercostal muscles between our ribs tighten. As they tighten, they do not allow our ribs to move as much as before, and this creates the sensation of wearing a corset around our thoracic (chest) region when we take that deep breath into the chest. This is why we feel that choking, restricted sensation when breathing in.

Endurance, or stamina, is the body's ability to perform better over a greater length of time with less stress and fatigue. By controlling the breath at the abdominals and expanding the lung capacity, you can achieve greater stamina. Many people think that only aerobic activity can increase stamina. However, deeper, controlled breathing, combined with even "low-grade," or nonaerobic, physical activity is also capable of increasing stamina. As you are able to achieve a certain level of exercise with ease, increase the repetitions without resting. Performing these over a period of time, with the same initial ease, will increase muscle endurance and tone.

After several weeks of following the this method, people who were previously not active have reported increased stamina when going for what was once a strenuous half-hour walk—in fact, a one-and-a-half-hour walk was not particularly demanding. Their muscle tone had increased, and with it their ability to walk a greater distance with less stress or strain also improved.

If you practice controlled, slow, deep breathing during exercising, you will become accustomed to breathing in this way, so that it will be-

come the norm even when you are at rest. This is not only less stressful on the body as a whole but can also lower your resting heart rate, which can be a determining factor in your longevity.

There are several ways to overcome the previously mentioned tightness in the chest. The following are two simple methods to assist in deeper breathing:

1. Repeat the sitting posture as above, with the hands pressed firmly below the navel. Now, instead of breathing into the chest, breathe "into your back." This concept may be difficult to grasp at first. If you find this difficult, try breathing into your shoulder blades (without rounding your shoulders, looking down, or collapsing your chest). This achieves the same result and more. You will find that after a few attempts, the breathing is deeper and the former, restricted breath into the chest has diminished a great deal. You may also find that, though you breathe more easily, your breath is still not going totally into the chest but more into the sides, under the arms. This is a good start to stretching those tight intercostals. Breathe in and out ten times, to a five-second count for the in breath and a five-second count for

CASE STUDY

Opera singers often feel uncomfortable about strengthening or tightening their stomach muscles. This is because they use the diaphragm to control their voice projection. But opera singers who have followed Pilates have felt that their singing actually improved because their abdominal control increased.

Over several months, as their stomach muscles improved and strengthened, the effect of "forcing" the deeper breathing into the lungs and chest cavity also stretched the intercostal muscles. With better abdominal strength, which they could now control, and increased lung capacity, they were able to hold notes for longer periods as well as use the previously barely existent abdominals for better voice projection.

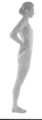

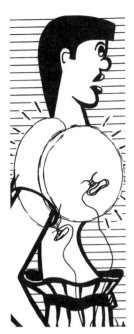

Figure 14. Breathing exercise "into your back"

the out breath. This will be the standard breathing method for the majority of the exercises in this book. So, whenever you feel a tight sensation as you breathe, remember to breathe into your back.

2.   The second method of attaining the correct breathing control and position is to kneel on the floor on your haunches with your chest on your thighs and your forehead resting on the floor, or on cushions if that is more comfortable. Place your hands as high up on your back, on the ribs, as you can without any tension in the neck or shoulder areas. In this position it would be fairly difficult to take a deep breath into the chest, as it is pressed against your thighs. Now breathe into your hands. This has the same effect as breathing into the back. Try not to breathe into the chest or the abdominal area. Practice these for ten breaths in and out.

General Breathing Rules

There are certain general breathing rules to follow when performing any of the movements. (There are always some exceptions to the rules, which I will point out as they occur.)

1. *When lying on the back (supine),* with the arms or the legs moving vertically away from the center, breathe *out.* When the arms or the legs move vertically toward the center, breathe *in.* At all times, *maintain the B-Line.*

2. *When the arm or legs move laterally (out to the sides)* away from the midline of the body, breathe *in.* For example, when performing "flies" (lying on the back and opening the arms outward with the arms to the ceiling, breathe *in* as the arms open out to the sides and breathe *out* as they come back to the center.

3. *When lying in the side position or on the stomach (prone),* if any part of the body is lifted against gravity, maintain the B-Line and breathe *out.* Breathe *in* when lowering to the floor.

4. *When on all fours (hands and feet/knees),* for most movements drawing away from the center or elongating the body, breathe *in.* When closing toward the center, keep the navel firmly to the spine and breathe *out.* For example, see Leg Pull Front (Exercise 54).

5. When contracting (curling forward) or rotating the torso, breathe *out.*

Exercise

Lie on your back on the floor with your knees bent and hands placed by your sides, palms upward. Extend one leg into the air and slowly lower this leg away from you, breathing out. (For those with stronger abdominals, try this exercise with both legs in the air.) The same can be done with the arms in the air, stretching them toward the floor above the head.

As you lower the arms or legs vertically away from your center, you may notice one of two things. You may actually want to breathe in, as it may feel unnatural to breathe out. In addition, as the arm or leg lowers to the floor, the lower back may have a tendency to arch. Be sure to maintain the B-Line when you feel this happening. You have gone as far as you are able to comfortably. Do not attempt to lower past this point. Greater abdominal control is required to lower the arm or leg farther without the back arching.

If you breathe in as you lower the arms or legs, not only does the lower back have a tendency to arch but the rib cage also has a tendency to poke up into the air.

Now breathe out as you extend the arms or legs away, and concentrate on keeping the back as flat as possible—flatten your rib cage as if a large weight had been placed on it. At the same time, to keep the back flat, press your abdominal muscles to the floor and feel them tighten. Imagine your arms or legs floating toward the floor. Can you

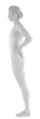

feel how this has a greater stabilizing effect on the spine? Can you feel how the abdominals and ribs work harder to maintain this position? Can you feel how your back is more supported without much stress on the spine?

4. CONTROL

Ideally, our muscles should obey our will. Reasonably, our will should not be dominated by the reflex actions of our muscles.

J. PILATES

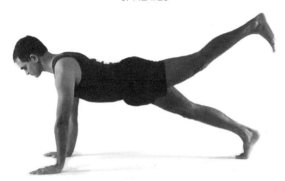

Breathe in on leg lift

Once the preceding principles have been practiced and mastered as best as possible, the next principle, that of control, can be more easily applied. Control is essential in preventing injuries. Maintaining control of every movement takes concentration, effort, and awareness of what the rest of the body is doing at the same time.

Whether the movements involve simply lengthening the neck and maintaining that position in order to reduce cervical lordosis (an arch in the neck), or a larger movement, such as a *grande ronde de jambe* in classical dance, the degree of control required may be the same. When someone initially practices these movements, it takes effort and concentration to perfect them to the best of the person's ability. Repetition, dedication, and application improve the degree of control and the perfection of the movement.

Uncontrolled, "automatic" movements, such as rapid lat pull-downs (behind the head pull-downs that engage the latissimus dorsi muscles) with weight equipment or the movements in some aerobics classes, can lead to injury if incorrect muscles are employed and incorrect posture is enforced. The action becomes mindless. Without concentration and control, the body's stronger muscles will tend to do all the work (and stay stronger) and the weaker, usually flabby muscles tend to remain relatively unused and therefore remain weak.

It is control over weaker parts of the body that improves their strength. Strength can also be improved in the major muscle groups (which may already have a certain degree of strength), by increasing the load on the muscle and attempting to maintain the same control over the movement as when the load was lighter. This is usually achieved by increasing the load by small amounts.

When muscles are in continual motion, they are being toned. When there is no control (no toning "connection"), they are underutilized. So, in broad terms, if you are not toning a muscle, you are "flabbing" it.

If you have difficulty mentally "feeling" the weak muscles, then follow this suggestion. Place your fingers into the weak / soft / flabby muscle to create a mental connection. For example, when performing Single Leg Circles 1 (Exercise 22), place your fingers into the inner thigh, as shown in Figure 15. Press the fingers against the muscle when taking the leg out to the side, and press the muscle against the fingers when drawing the leg to the center. This will give your mind a better connection to the muscle you really want to work, rather than the quadriceps (thigh) muscle, which you might otherwise tend to overwork.

Control does not necessarily mean a reduction in performance. Initially, as you learn to gain control while doing a certain movement, some performance may be compromised. But when you have perfected the movement, the greater control will allow you to do it more quickly and

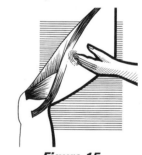

Figure 15. Fingers in muscle

exceed your previous levels of performance.

5. PRECISION

Correctly executed and mastered to the point of subconscious reaction, these exercises will reflect grace and balance in your routine activities.

J. PILATES

Precision of movement leads to more graceful movements. We see this with classical ballet dancers, who are required to fine-tune their bodies in order to achieve an exactness of a simple, or even complex, series of jumps, *ports de bras,* or *plies,* as well as in gymnasts, who require perfect balance and control when performing on the balance beam or parallel bars. When all these movements are performed in a group, as in synchronized swimming, we can see the beauty, grace, style, and apparent effortlessness that is the result of the precise actions of the participants.

Precision requires thought (back to that essential principle of concentration) and mental feedback (visualizing and understanding what the perfect movement is). Our bodies require this feedback to let us know that we are achieving results. It is usually very difficult to obtain this feedback when working weaker muscle groups, because the stronger ones tend to take on most of the workload.

Precision of movement can be accomplished in short actions, such as when a weight trainer lifts a heavy weight or a bodybuilder performs on stage. Precision requires controlled action, without which the movement becomes sloppy and aesthetically unappealing. The space within which you move and perform various physical activities also determines, and is determined by, precision.

This is very obviously seen in comparing a gymnast performing on a balance beam to the same gymnast performing a floor routine. One performance is very confined and restricted (closed physical movement), the other very open and generally unrestricted (open physical movement). Both, however, require precision to achieve

the goals required. Precision also requires correct positioning prior to beginning the movement to attain better performance.

Precision of movement not only requires correct placement of the body before commencing an exercise, but also regulating the speed with which the movement is performed in relation to other parts of the body and the breathing. For example, if an exercise requires the movement of your arm above the head as you breathe out, the movement should be synchronized so that the last part of the exhalation coincides with the reach of the arm above the head. If more breath is expelled at the beginning of the movement, so that you are holding your breath for the last 20 percent of the arm's travel, precision of movement is not achieved. The exercise then becomes stressful rather than flowing and coordinated.

6. FLOWING MOVEMENT

Contrology® is designed to give you suppleness, natural grace and skill that will be unmistakably reflected in [all you do].

J. PILATES

Fluidity of movement while exercising leads to fluidity of movement when not exercising. Conscious muscular control through all ranges of movement will help eliminate stiff, jerky movements. It is in the extreme ranges of movement (ROM) that less control is likely to occur, as muscles tend to be weaker in elongated positions. As a result, there is less flowing movement.

For example, when you extend a leg or an arm to kick or punch, the fast movement at the extremity (end of range) can produce a "snapping" effect in the knee or elbow joint. Continuous repetitions of this action can result in pain in the joint. This snapping of the joint is also an indication that the muscles are not in as complete control as you might think.

This sharp movement can, and should, be eliminated to reduce any long-term wearing effect on the joint. If it is caused by hyperextension of the joint, then extension should be done only to the point where the joint is "unlocked" (not noticeably bent). To a person with hyperextension, the joint would feel quite bent. However, from a normal visual approach, the limbs would appear straight.

Stiff movements also occur in muscles that are too tight. We often see this with bodybuilders who lift extremely heavy weights. They walk with short, restricted movements. Their biceps muscles are so tight that their arms are continuously bent, giving the appearance of a gorilla's arm posture. Fluid movement may initially require a shortening of overextended muscles and a lengthening of the tight ones.

Make your movements continuous, rather than stopping for even a fraction of a second. Continue the movements as if ten repetitions were one, rather than one repetition repeated ten times.

7. ISOLATION

Each muscle may cooperatively and loyally aid in the uniform development of all our muscles.
J. PILATES

Once you have gained control of a weaker muscle group, you can achieve even more control over that muscle group as well as increased isolation. Enhanced precision of movement is then also possible.

Attempt this movement, for example: Lie on your back, keeping your arms slightly bent at the elbow with the palm of the hand facing the floor. Now attempt to isolate and tighten the triceps muscle (the muscles in the back of the upper arm) of your weaker arm. Do not straighten the arm, hunch the shoulder, clench the fist, or make the forearm become rigid. Do not press the arm onto the floor. (For those of you with good body awareness and physical conditioning, this may not be too difficult, so attempt the same with the hamstring of the weaker leg, the lower abdominals, the weaker rhomboid, or some other weaker part of the body.)

Can you feel the triceps tighten?

For many of you it may be quite difficult to engage that triceps muscle, let alone feel where it is. The first response is to use all of the negative muscular reactions to feel the contraction of the triceps. Some of you may be confounded that you cannot feel anything at all!

Now, touch the triceps with gentle pressure with your other hand, and tighten the triceps. The reaction this time may be instantaneous. The connection is made. The physical contact, or touch response, provides the simple biofeedback necessary to make the mental/physical connection possible. Without the touch response, it was difficult to obtain a good connection of the muscle or even to identify where the muscle was located. Now, take this a step further. Press the triceps with more force, as if you were pressing the bone of the humerus (upper arm) itself. Now tighten the triceps. The reaction of the muscle is even better.

The increase in pressure usually results in a better response, because we are attempting to work from the core of the muscle itself. This increase in receptivity of the muscle function usually leads to faster results than if the muscle were not being touched at all.

If you are unable to obtain the connection, do not despair. It may take several, or even many, attempts for the muscle to respond. This is usually a result of not working the muscle often enough. Generally, the stronger muscle groups will do the majority of the work in any movement. Concentration alone may not be enough to fire those receptors to engage the weaker muscles that require toning or strength. You may need to use the touch response for several weeks on the same muscle before having even the slightest reaction. A muscle does not need to hurt or be sore the next day for you to know that it is working. The firmness of the muscle, or the speed with which it responds, is a good indication that it is working well.

Once you have gained better control over the weaker muscle, the physical contact is no longer required to "feel" the muscle working. With isolation comes flexibility of the limb, lever, or joint. If we can isolate a part of the body and allow it to move independently of other parts, we are in a better position to introduce more flexibility to that area (assuming we have only muscular, and not structural/bony, restrictions).

Flexibility is defined as "the range of movement of a specific joint or group of joints influenced by the associated bones and bony structures and the physiological characteristics of the muscles, tendons, ligaments, and various other collagenous tissues surrounding the joint" (Arnheim, *Modern Principles of Athletic Training*).

Combining all of the principles we have discussed so far can lead to increased flexibility of the joints and better physical performance. Further means of achieving flexibility, such as specific muscle stretching techniques, can also lead to

greater results. I have devoted an entire section to flexibility and stretching, as this is extremely important in the prevention of injuries (see "The Warm-Up," pp. 58–70).

Too much flexibility can lead to loss of muscular control, and too little can restrict movement—both conditions can lead to injury. As an example of the former, classical ballet dancers are generally thought to be extremely flexible. However, many of them would like to have more strength in the extreme ranges of movement without compromising their flexibility or building bulk. At the other end of the spectrum, triathletes tend to feel they are too tight and would certainly like to have more flexibility, without compromising their strength, and thereby achieve better times.

8. ROUTINE

Patience and persistence are vital qualities in the ultimate successful accomplishment of any worthwhile endeavor.

J. PILATES

Establishing a regular routine, whether it is daily or three times a week, can undoubtedly lead to greater results. Many people ask, "How long will it take me to get fit?" or "How often should I exercise?" The answer is relative to the person asking the question. Would you like to become as fit as your next-door neighbor, who may not consider himself fit at all? Or do you go by some other standard?

An established Pilates routine will improve mental and physical conditioning in all individuals. The more you do, the better the result.

A simple analogy would be playing the piano. To most of us this would seem a daunting task. But even the world's maestros started from scratch. Their perseverance, dedication, energy, and regular practice made them what they are. The same applies to all activities. One practice session a week will achieve far less than two, three, or four a week. The more you do, the better the result. Your sense of well-being will be vastly improved, and you will see the world through different eyes.

The workout, including stretches, should last between 1 and 1¼ hours. Doing two workout sessions per week to start is a good effort. Three workouts per week is excellent! The gradual im-

provement as you master the exercises will build your confidence in what you are able to achieve physically. This system of muscle conditioning, of combining the focused mental concentration with the physical aspects I have described, can produce a lean, defined, muscularly balanced physique. I often tell clients to think of this not as exercise (especially when they blow their breath out through pursed lips) but simply as movement. Movement that is fluid, unforced, but precise and controlled. Don't be surprised if you do not see much of a result for up to two months. As mentioned earlier, the method works from the inside out. To engage muscles that you never knew even existed takes time. On the other hand, you may be surprised at how soon the results appear!

When performing the exercises, imagine that they are everyday movements, not enforced exercises. Imagine the improved control these movements can then induce in even your normal activities. Imagine walking up stairs and feeling your hamstrings firmly in control. Imagine picking up a baby and feeling your abdominal muscles supporting your back, or even lifting an object from an awkward position and feeling in total control of all the fibers in your body. All without having to think about these connections happening!

This is what Pilates is all about: improved quality of movement that can lead to an improved quality of life. Your life is in your hands. Grasp it with enthusiasm and change the way you think, feel, and react to all around you.

CHAPTER 3

The Importance of Posture

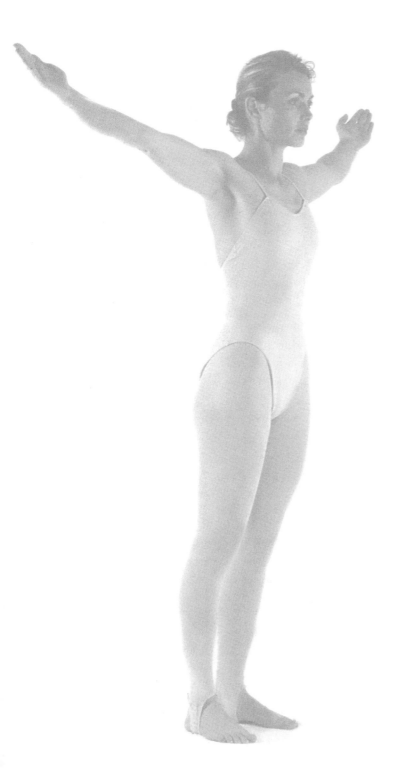

Contrology® develops
the body uniformly,
corrects wrong postures,
restores physical vitality,
invigorates the mind, and
elevates the spirit.

J. PILATES

any people think of posture and physique as interdependent. But it is not necessarily true that the better your physique, the better your posture.

BODY TYPES

According to the Sheldon classification, there are three basic human types:

1. *Endomorph:* larger than average, with soft, large abdomen and high shoulders.

2. *Ectomorph:* thin muscles and small bones, with drooped shoulders.

3. *Mesomorph:* large thorax, slender waist, thick abdominal muscles.

The average person lies between the ectomorph and the mesomorph.

FACTORS INFLUENCING POSTURE

Any of the body types can have good or bad posture. Adult posture is more inclined to be dependent on the following:

■ *Inherited conditions:* genetic makeup determines an individual's height, type of bone structure, and so on.

■ *Habit:* from occupational or repetitive movements, muscle function becomes restrictive, altering postural alignment.

■ *Disease:* whether muscular or structural (as in bone deformity), disease certainly alters one's stance, and limitations are then imposed on one's normal activity.

I have already discussed the effects of gravity on the muscles. They are constantly being pulled downward. Our bodies are required to counter these forces with healthy, strong muscle structures to maintain good posture and ward off the effects of strain and injury.

WHAT IS CORRECT POSTURE?

In order to discuss postural deviation, we need to understand what is meant by normal posture. To do this, imagine a plumb line going through your body when you are standing upright:

1. From the side (lateral) view, the plumb line should pass from the top of your skull through the center of your body to the floor, through your center of gravity. It passes through the ear lobe, the center of the tip of the shoulder, the hip joint, behind the patella of the knee, and midway between the heel and the balls of the foot.

2. From the back (posterior) view, the plumb line should fall through the center of the scull, following the line of the spine, the hips (between the cheeks of the buttocks), and on to the floor with the lower limbs equally placed on either side of the line, and the knees and heels directly below the hips. The knees, pelvis, and shoulders should also be parallel to the floor.

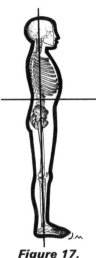

Figure 17. Correct posture

Your center of gravity should lie along the intersection of these two lines and a third line, which is found in the section between your hips and your lower ribs.

THE TRIPOD POSITION

To achieve overall balance of the body in a standing position, you should make sure that the feet evenly support the body when they are placed directly under the hip joints. The body's weight should be evenly distributed over the three points that form a triangle on the feet: (1) the ball of the big toe, (2) the outside edge of the foot, and (3) the center of the heel. There should be no pressure forward on the toes or backward on the heels. By also placing an equal pressure on the outside edge of the foot, you

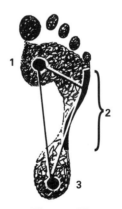

Figure 18. The Tripod Position

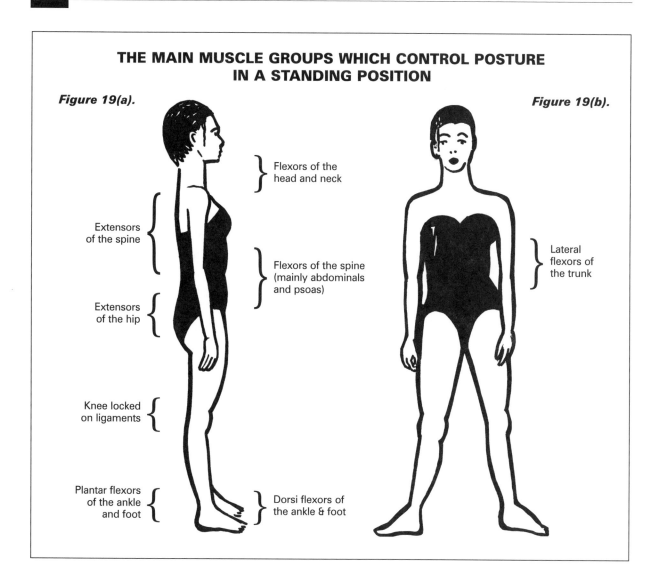

THE MAIN MUSCLE GROUPS WHICH CONTROL POSTURE IN A STANDING POSITION

Figure 19(a).

Figure 19(b).

Flexors of the head and neck

Extensors of the spine

Flexors of the spine (mainly abdominals and psoas)

Extensors of the hip

Lateral flexors of the trunk

Knee locked on ligaments

Plantar flexors of the ankle and foot

Dorsi flexors of the ankle & foot

may feel as if you are creating an arch where the arch should be. Try to maintain this tripod position whenever standing.

POSTURAL ASSESSMENT

Correct posture may be determined either by visual means or by actual measurement, when the eye cannot detect slight misalignments. The following are two main areas where the posture can deviate from the norm:

1. The lower limbs: feet, tibia/fibula, and femur.

2. The pelvis and torso: the pelvis and the lumbar, thoracic, and cervical sections of the spine and rib cage.

Bad posture in the lower limbs can result from conditions such as the following:

1. Foot pronation or supination, inversion or eversion.

   a) Knock knees (genu valgum) and bow legs (genu varum).

   b) Hyperextended or hyperflexed knees.

   c) Leg length differences.

   d) Tibial torsion (when the feet are parallel and the knees roll in).

   The first two and the fourth can be detected from a front view and the third from a side view.

2. Pelvic and spinal alignment

a) Anterior (forward) or posterior (back-ward) tilt of the pelvis.

b) Lumbar lordosis.

c) Kyphosis.

d) Cervical lordosis.

e) Scoliosis.

3. Actions of the scapula (shoulder blade) and shoulder such as the following:

a) Elevation: hunched shoulders.

b) Depression: pushed down shoulders.

c) Adduction: shoulders squeezed together.

d) Abduction: winged shoulder blades.

e) Forward rotation of the shoulders.

Side viewing can detect positions a through d), while viewing from the back can detect position e).

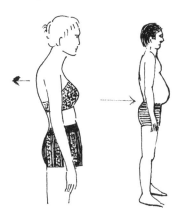

Figure 20.
Kyphosis   Lordosis

BAD POSTURE AND LOWER BACK PAIN

The following is a common example of how bad posture can affect the lower back. Simply stand with your hands on your hips. This simple, seemingly innocent movement has no fewer than four detrimental effects on the body.

You will notice that the hands are usually placed with the fingers on the front of the hips and the thumbs hooked at the top of the hipbones at the back. Most people adopt this stance, especially if they have lower back pain. Others may

adopt the "pregnancy" stance by placing the hands in the small of the back and pushing forward, creating a large arch in the lower back. In the long term, both stances, especially the pregnancy stance, cause the following in most individuals:

The pelvis tilts forward, leading to

1. Arching of the lower back, which causes these muscles to become shorter and tighter.

2. Shortening of the thigh muscles, which draws the pelvis farther forward, "locking" the hips. This is commonly seen in men with beer guts who are unable to tilt the pelvis backward.

3. Loosening and stretching of the lower abdominals.

4. Hunching of the shoulders, leading to tighter neck muscles.

Figure 21.
Pregnancy
stance

MUSCLE IMBALANCES

Muscles that overwork or strain on a frequent basis can generally cause an imbalance of the skeletal structure. It is commonly assumed that overworked muscles need stretching and underworked muscles require strengthening for the body to be in a position of balance or equilibrium. Postural defects that can be corrected are those that are created by weak or overstrong muscles. More than just muscle reconditioning is required to alleviate structural problems, and indeed, to correct the posture.

The hip flexors have an enormous effect on the body's structure, especially its posture. The psoas major and iliacus, if overstrong, tend to lift or lurch the body from a flat (supine) position to sitting upright.

In order to roll the spine into an upright position, these hip flexors need to be controlled by producing more mid- and lower abdominal strength.

Another group of hip flexors is the quadriceps or thigh muscles. There are four (Latin, *quad*) major groups of muscles in the thigh. They attach from the top of the hip and femur to the patella

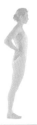

and quadriceps tendon. As they are the largest group of muscles in the body, they tend to do a great deal of work without any conscious effort involved. From when we are babies, with our legs in the air, to the time we crawl, to the time we stand erect to walk, run, or jump, the thigh muscles are continuously engaged.

Continually exposing these muscles to overexertion without opposite relief, such as stretching, can cause problems such as back pain.

When the muscles of the upper thigh are overstrong they tend to tilt the pelvis in an anterior position. This, in turn, tends to create a small arch in the lower back, lengthening the lower abdominals and causing the iliopsoas hip flexors to also shorten and accentuate the arch in the small of the back. Although the mid- and upper abdominals may appear flat, they may not be working hard enough to counter the strength of the hip flexors pulling the spine forward. This imbalance can cause considerable back pain.

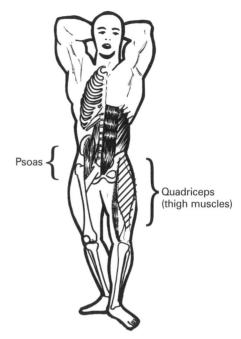

Psoas

Quadriceps (thigh muscles)

Figure 22. The hip flexors

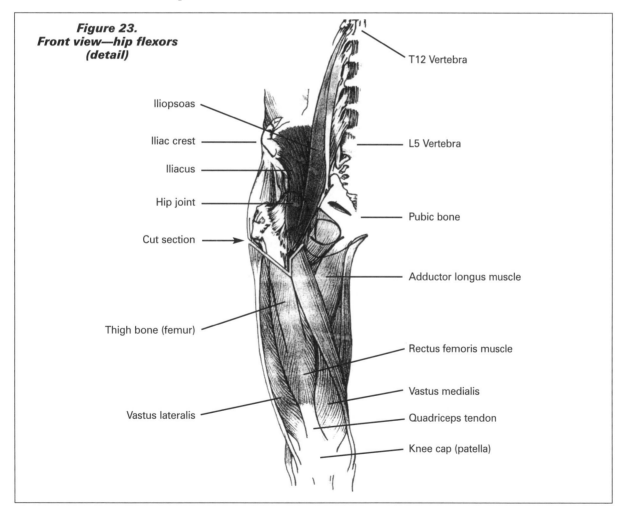

Figure 23. Front view—hip flexors (detail)

Iliopsoas

Iliac crest

Iliacus

Hip joint

Cut section

Thigh bone (femur)

Vastus lateralis

T12 Vertebra

L5 Vertebra

Pubic bone

Adductor longus muscle

Rectus femoris muscle

Vastus medialis

Quadriceps tendon

Knee cap (patella)

CASE STUDY

A sixteen-year-old female, with a previous history of ballet and, more recently, gymnastics, saw her practitioner for mild, but increasing, lower back pain. The patient's physique was that of a fit young girl with no postural deviations and flat abdominals. Upon examination by X-ray and CAT scans, it was discovered that there was a mild posterior disc bulge at L4-5. The pain gradually became worse, with no alleviation of the symptoms from various forms of practitioner treatment. Her movements were akin to that of a fifty-year-old with severe back pain.

When the client came to the studio, it was discovered that her trunk hip flexors were doing all the work, and she had only minimal abdominal strength. Manual pressure was applied to the lower abdominals at the psoas level and lower limb activity was undertaken, which reduced the pain levels. Lower abdominal work, especially focusing on the B-Line, was initiated. The woman's condition improved approximately 10 percent over four months. After twelve months of treatment in a studio situation, using equipment, the condition improved 80 percent. There are now only occasional setbacks in the client's progress.

In general, we can equate back pain to a lack of muscle strength in a corresponding section of the abdominal area and, in some cases, a combination of other tight muscle groups. The above is a generalization, and situations will vary from case to case. As we can see, certain imbalances are not visually noticeable, but, although the posture appears normal, the effects are considerable.

As described above, a tightening of the thigh muscles can lead to an arching of the lower back. As this continues, the lower back and psoas muscles also become contracted, and the latter draw the lumbar vertebra forward. This creates stress on the spinal column and the discs in between. This pressure, caused by a combination of tight back, psoas, and thigh muscles, can exert enough pressure on the spine to squeeze nerves between the disc and the vertebra, resulting in sciatic pain.

From this common example above, we can recognize the fact that muscles work in conjunction with each other. A chain reaction can occur when misalignment of muscles in one part of the body causes the need for a compensation in another part, farther up or down the line. In the above example, a further compensation for the hyperextension in the lower back (lumbar vertebrae) could be a tendency to sway back at the knees.

IDENTIFYING PAIN

Injuries occur even in people who are fit or think they are fit. When an injury occurs, other muscles take over some of the work to alleviate the pressure on the injured area. As a result, some of these muscles exert themselves more than they have done in the past. As they become stronger they too then tend to pull the body further out of alignment. So, once the injury has been resolved, another problem has occurred that requires correcting. Muscle wastage (or atrophy) is common in sports and other types of injuries. Although the person thinks he is fit, he may still be in pain owing to increased pressure on the limbs or joints from other muscles that have been automatically recruited to keep the structure functioning as normally as possible.

There are three areas where, during the exercise routine, you should never feel any pressure, strain, or pain:

1. The back.

2. The neck.

3. Any of the other joints.

Although the neck and back are also joints, I have itemized them separately here for easier identification by those new to discovering their bodies through movement.

If you continue to participate in sports while still feeling pain in certain movements, you should first take appropriate action to determine what the pain is and employ clinical efforts (treatment, scans, etc.) to alleviate the problem. If the pain still persists, before beginning an exercise program it is essential to take the following steps:

1. Identify the area of pain: muscle, joint, tissue, or bone.

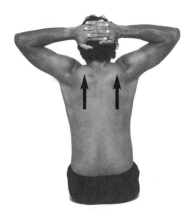

Figure 24(a). Incorrect

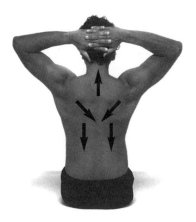

Figure 24(b). Correct

2. Assess the level of pain during the specific movements (for instance, is pain present only when the activity takes place?).

3. Determine the amount of restriction of the painful area.

4. Determine whether the area has suffered a previous injury or trauma.

5. Establish whether scar tissue is present that would restrict the full range of motion.

Joint Strains

Joint strains are fairly common and can be corrected quite easily in the early stages. If there is any strain in any joint when exercising, it is important to do the following:

1. Reduce the range of movement of the joint.

2. If the strain persists, reduce the rotation of the joint (if externally or internally rotated at the joint).

3. If the strain is in a hinge joint (knee/elbow), reduce the extension or flexion at the hinge.

4. If the strain is in the rotating joint and the hinge joint is hyperextended, bend the hinge joint to better engage the muscle between the rotating joint and the hinge joint (you might try a single leg circle with the hand on the knee, as in Exercise 22).

Neck Strain

Neck strain during exercising can, in most cases, be alleviated by following these steps:

1. Draw the scapulae toward each other and then to the hip line without arching the back.

2. Lengthen the neck (reducing any lordosis), as in Figure 24(b).

3. If the strain persists when exercising on your back, place a comfortable cushion under the head (not too high, as this will not help alleviate the condition). Keep the head rested during the exercise.

Lower Back Strain

Lower back strain during exercising is generally caused by the back arching or hyperextending. Try the following to alleviate lower back strain:

1. Flatten the back by imprinting the spine onto the floor and then doing the B-Line. (If standing, imagine you are standing against a wall or actually stand against a wall with your feet six inches away from the wall.)

2. If your back is still arched, do some thigh stretches (see Exercises 11 to 13) to mobilize the hip joints. This may alleviate the problem almost immediately for a short period of time, but it must be continued on a regular basis.

3. Tilt the pelvis under slightly (posterior tilt) to correct the arch. If lying down, do not lift the hips off the floor.

4. If you are lying down with the knees bent and the back is still arched, then draw the knees to the chest.

5. If standing, draw the rib cage to the imaginary wall, without rounding the shoulders, and bend the knees.

THE STRETCH PAIN AND WORK SCALES

When following an exercise or stretching routine, it is important to listen to what your body is telling you. The myth of "No pain, no gain" is old-fashioned and dangerous. The "burn" or pain you feel could actually be microfiber tears of the muscle itself!

A certain amount of soreness is acceptable if you have not worked out for some time and decide to engage in even a mild circuit class. It is best, in these cases, to do a correctly executed stretching routine before the start of a class or partake in a mild stretch class the next day to alleviate any aches and pains from the previous day.

Stretching of the muscles should be performed gradually, and, if an uncomfortable level of pain occurs the next day, it may be an indication of excessive muscular work. Ease up on the regime and the situation should correct itself. Continual working and stretching through pain is not an intelligent approach to good body maintenance. The muscles need time to repair themselves before further exertion is applied to them. In the long term, this could lead to those niggling, recurring complaints that can haunt you for years. If you do have this problem, consult a trained, exercise-oriented health care professional or a qualified Pilates instructor.

Naturally, a certain amount of pain will occur during training, even after proper warming up. In order to challenge ourselves to become better at any physical activity we intend to undertake, a certain pain level is acceptable. The real question is, Up to what level is this pain acceptable? In any case, if the pain is sudden, sharp, uncomfortable, or acute, our body is telling us that we must cease that activity.

While exercising, it may be useful to adopt the following Stretch Pain Scale guideline to assess your pain levels. This guide is in a very simple format and is intended to be used only to monitor "normal" pain levels. If any unusual twinges or momentarily sharp pain occurs, reduce the exercise or stretch to a level that is comfortable.

The Stretch Pain Scale is a simple scale of zero to ten, zero being where no stretch occurs and no pain is felt. Ten, on the other hand, is where the pain level is extremely uncomfortable and unbearable. The position cannot be maintained. This is a level where you feel there is no benefit to your body. Regularly striving for this level may result in long-term tissue damage and is to be avoided at all costs. (The only exceptions to this rule are the Thigh Stretches, Exercises 11 to 13.)

- **1–5**: If you feel any pain or discomfort during a movement or stretch, ask yourself at what level this is. If it lies between levels 1 and 5, then you may feel that a mild stretch and continued stretching in this zone is safe (taking into account that no other parts of the body are being affected).

- **6–8**: If the strong stretch is between levels 6 and 8, you will experience a strong muscular stretch but no pain. This stretch has a beneficial muscular feeling to it, and you know that you are able to maintain the position comfortably. This has a "doing you

Figure 25.

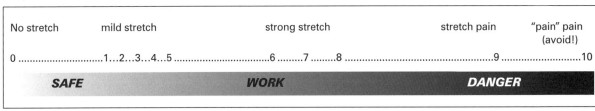

No stretch	mild stretch		strong stretch		stretch pain	"pain" pain (avoid!)
0 ....1...2...3...4...5 ....6 ....7 ....8 ....9 10

| SAFE | WORK | DANGER |

Graph I.

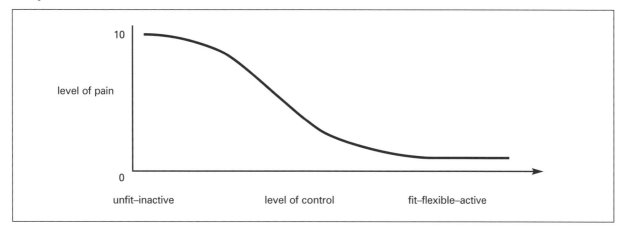

level of pain

10

0

unfit–inactive   level of control   fit–flexible–active

good" feel to it. You know you are really doing some work. You are being challenged at this level.

- **9**: When approaching level 9, the feel of the stretch or movement changes from one of comfort to one of discomfort and pain. In this zone, damage may occur. It is better to back off from this level of exercise rather than risking forcing the muscles and possibly causing injury.

- **10**: Level 10 is unbearable pain and should never be experienced.

Only very experienced athletes who understand their bodies through many years of training (and, usually, many injuries) would be able to continue working in what to most of us is the danger zone, with any benefit. The body awareness of athletes of this caliber is heightened, not only by the stringent demands they make on their bodies but also by the mental discipline that their regimes require to attain the best result.

The Work Scale, on the other hand, involves muscular control. It, too, is on a scale of zero to ten.

- **0**: No work at all.

- **1–5**: The exercise can be easily controlled. Many repetitions can be performed at this level.

- **6–9**: Exercise at this level is an increasing challenge.

- **10**: The exercise cannot be controlled.

The Stretch Pain Scale always dictates. What this means is that if the Stretch Pain Scale is 8 and the Work Scale is only 3, for that particular exercise, the 8 level is to be observed. Do not push the Work Scale to attain its challenge range (6–9). This will only push the Stretch Pain Scale further! As the stretching routines continue on a regular basis, the Stretch Pain Scale may ease back to 6 or so. In this case, the Work Scale can then be increased to 4 or 5, and so on.

BODY POSITIONING FOR BETTER EXERCISING

Before beginning an exercise regime or a specific exercise, it is essential to assume the correct posture or position in order to connect the correct muscle groups. When you assume the correct posture, your energy is focused on the muscles that require it and not wasted on other areas or on unnecessary movements.

This is especially true when beginning an exercise that is totally new to your body. New exercise programs generally require concentration and control to which the body may never have been subjected.

For instance, suppose a triathlete has never attempted a yoga class before. The new positions require a great deal of thought and focus. Muscles are being subjected to movements that are new to them, and forcing these movements can cause injury, especially as the positions are held for some time. It is always important to keep in mind that any new routine for the body must be approached with caution.

Because triathletes are quite fit compared to the general population, they also approach physical challenges more readily and sometimes throw themselves into new regimes with the mental attitude that their bodies can endure any new venture. Such an athlete may not spend an hour stretching.

The muscles, however, have memorized only certain movements as a result of countless hours of repeating those movements over many years. Once the body and mind have approached a routine in a certain manner, it is difficult to change that pattern without changes to the result. These changes may initially be adverse—such as slower times or shorter jumping distances—until the muscles accept their new regime as the set basis upon which to progress.

Our bodies will invariably take the easy way out. They will perform movements that require the least effort and concentration. When we are not focused, our bodies will cheat on us! To illustrate this, lie on your back with your arms extended to the ceiling above your chest. This may be done with or without hand weights. Make sure your arms are not above your face or neck, but directly above the chest in line with the shoulders. Keeping them in line with the shoulders, slowly open the arms out to the sides (to the floor) and then close them to the ceiling again. Repeat this half a dozen times. Notice that as you do more repetitions, the arms slowly start to move above the face when in the air and in line with the head when open to the floor. This has the effect of gradually raising the shoulders with the neck muscle engaged. Imagine the effect when the exercise is repeated hundreds of times!

To work specific muscle groups requires concentration and effort. To maintain an almost perfect regime of such movements, until they form the required engram so the movement becomes automatic, requires a pattern for muscular development and achievement for that movement.

To accomplish this, you need to establish a routine. Once you have achieved this, then any new movements, such as an attempt at yoga when you've previously been a triathlete, can be approached safely. You can perform your own "self-check" as to the requirements, benefits, limits, and dangers to which your body will be exposed.

ESTABLISHING A PATTERN FOR MUSCULAR CONTROL

I have developed a formula that will help you perform an exercise to the best of your physical ability, no matter what your level of fitness.

At first, it may seem difficult to follow all the points of the formula at the same time. However, by systematically covering each part sequentially, and mastering that principle before the next is undertaken, you can perfect the exercise and develop good technique.

The formula, P/A/P, B, B, E, E, Q, refers to the following:

- Posture/Alignment/Position

- Back

- Breathing

- Exercise

- Elongation

- Questions

The formula has been designed to help you make each exercise precise and gain the most benefit out of each movement or series of movements. A gradual approach to a new routine will establish a solid foundation to use as a springboard in developing greater speed, range, or control in the movement or routine.

It has been found that if this formula is adhered to, it is almost impossible to perform a routine incorrectly, or for an instructor to devise an incorrect movement for a client.

1. Posture/Alignment/Position

When beginning an exercise, it is important to establish the correct position or alignment for the exercise. If this is not correct from the start, the movement can become sloppy and less effective. This is especially important for rehabilitation exercise programs. Establishing and maintaining the correct position of a limb, the pelvis, or torso is crucial to the final outcome. A difference of one centimeter in an exercise can mean a difference of 10, 20, 30, 40, or even 50 percent in the effectiveness of the exercise. Imagine a gymnast on the parallel bars or on the beam who moves one centimeter off her projected alignment. She may lose

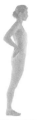

control or balance, or even worse, fall off the apparatus. Or if a tennis player misses the "sweet spot" on the racquet more times than his opponent, it could mean the difference between winning and losing, between perfection and "close enough is good enough." The same is true in developing the type of body you really want.

Training the brain to search for these small differences requires assistance. A mirror can help you to identify major differences in position and alignment.

The following are some questions to ask when practicing this principle of the formula. Keep in mind that this list is not exhaustive.

1. Are the hips square?

2. Is the leg in line with the shoulder?

3. Is the torso upright?

4. Is the foot flexed?

5. Are the shoulders level?

6. Is the back straight?

7. Is the stomach flat?

8. Is the neck elongated?

9. Are the shoulders relaxed?

2. Back

Ensure that the back is in the required position for the start of the exercise. Generally, when you are lying supine, the back should be as flat as possible, in the B-Line. It is important to "zip up" the B-Line. What is meant by this? Imagine you are trying to get into a very tight pair of jeans. Many of us have tried this before. We either lie on the bed or floor or bend ourselves over double to pull our stomachs in! Well, imagine you are doing this now. The lower abdominals are in the B-Line prior to starting the movement of the zipper. Then you need to maintain the B-Line as the zipper is closed all the way up, and imagine the B-Line coming up with the zipper.

This may be one of the few times many of us actually feel our lower abdominals contracting! This attempted, continual connection helps to strengthen this group of abdominal muscles. Strength in these lower abdominals greatly as-

sists in the relief of lower back pain and in the ability to tuck the pelvis under.

Control of the rib cage also provides stability for the spine (see the section that follows on breathing). When we are upright, is the back straight or is there a lean to one side? Is the lower back arched or the upper back too rounded? Is the head tilted forward or backward?

All these can be corrected to a certain extent by realignment and reeducation of the muscles. If the problem is more structural, as in some cases of osteoporosis, the spine and back should be aligned as best as possible, without causing any discomfort.

3. Breathing

Breathing has been covered in another section under the same heading. However, the manner of instruction for breathing is important and cannot be stressed too often.

When performing challenging small movements, many people hold their breath. As I mentioned earlier, it is important not to hold the breath while exercising. If you hold your breath while performing a movement, you will strain your body.

It is generally accepted that one should breathe out on the effort. For example, imagine you are doing a bodybuilding exercise, lying on your back on a low bench, lifting a heavy weight and working the triceps. To perform this movement, you extend both arms above the head and return them to the vertical position. There are several problems with this action.

This movement is usually done with the feet on the ground, creating an arch in the lower back before the exercise has even begun. This, in itself, can cause stress to the lower back and certainly a tightening of those muscles. When the weight lifter extends the arms overhead to the vertical position, the back is arched even farther as the pectorals almost lock past a certain point. There is limited mobility at the shoulder joint. The weight lifter usually takes a short breath in as the arms extend above the head and a heavy blow out as they are drawn back to the starting position, with a great deal of straining of the entire torso.

To control the exercise and work on the specific muscle group in a more focused manner, other areas of stress and strain should be elimi-

nated as much as possible. The breathing is usually one of these stress points. If the bodybuilder were to breathe as calmly as possible and still perform the exercise in whatever manner he wished, the exercise would look very easy; to those around him he would not appear to be working hard at all. The bodybuilder might need to lighten the weight to gain more control, because the different method of breathing would change their ability to perform the movement as they were used to doing previously.

If the weight lifter were to perform the same exercise with calmer breathing, a flatter back, and less facial expression, everyone would wonder what sort of super athlete this could be, displaying such control and ease of movement.

Breathing plays an important role in helping the body to cope with stress, whether mental or physical.

Often, when people are instructed to breathe during exercise, they are told something like this: "Lift your leg and breathe out." The message the mind has received is to move the limb and, at the completion of the movement, breathe out. In an exercise routine, the breathing instruction should ideally be phrased like this: "Breathe in (or out) as you…." Breathe for the duration of the movement to reduce stresses and strains, thereby avoiding injury. Breathe calmly in through the nose and sigh out through the mouth.

As you become accustomed to breathing in the manner appropriate for the movement, you can do faster repetitions, still breathing in normally for two, three, or four repetitions and out for the next two, three, or four. Controlled, calm breathing can certainly enhance physical performance.

4. Exercise

When you get to this point, you are performing the exercise as perfectly as possible. If you are unable to perfect the exercise with the correct breathing in the first half dozen movements, do not despair. Practice the exercise with whatever breathing feels comfortable at the time. Get the body to move and understand what is required of it. As this becomes more feasible and familiar, then adjust the breathing to the correct requirements.

Even when performing advanced exercises, return to the basic versions every so often. You will find that they, too, can be difficult to perform as more focus and connection is applied to the simpler movements.

5. Elongation

When moving the limbs or any part of the body, you can gain a greater feeling of working all muscles, especially the unused, smaller ones, by lengthening through the movement. For example, when standing or lying on your back, maintain a B-Line and keep the ribs lengthened away from the hips, while also pressing the shoulder blades to the hips. This requires more abdominal contraction and helps to keep the spine long and more flexible, as well as alleviating pressure on the vertebrae and discs.

When working on lengthening the arms or legs, do not lock the knee or elbow joints. This can cause stress on those joints. If these joints are hyperextended, then the bones are merely being locked together and the muscles will strain rather than work. You should also avoid too much of a bend, because that will not allow the muscle to lengthen and will restrict mobility of the limb from the socket. With the joint unlocked it is still possible to lengthen out of the socket (without moving the hip or shoulder) to attain the mobility required.

Continual lengthening of the muscle group being worked tends to have several distinct advantages. The following are some of the benefits gained from muscle lengthening:

- Leaner muscles, less bulk.

- Reduced stress on the joint.

- Increased awareness of specific, isolated muscle movement.

- Increased mobility of the joint.

- Reduced "clicking" of the joint.

The muscle group you wish to lengthen should initially be stable and injury-free. Lengthening of injured muscles can place more load on the fibers and lead to further problems.

In many exercise routines, especially those involving heavy weights, it is common for the limb to be unable to move through its full range. The body keeps the limb from extending to reduce the

amount of stress on the joint. However, not extending the muscle through its full range has the effect of shortening that muscle. In biceps curls, when lifting a heavy weight, the arm is rarely extended close to its full length. The upper body is also usually curled forward in order to prepare it to take the strain of the next lift. This movement, when the weight touches the thigh, gives the illusion that the arm has performed a close to full extension.

If the exercise were to be performed correctly through the full range with the same amount of effort, the weight would need to be reduced, because the biceps muscle fiber is weaker when almost fully extended. Once greater strength is achieved in the extended position, then an increased weight can be safely applied.

Similarly, in the abdominal curl, if the knees are bent at an acute angle at the knee joint (heels too close to the bottom), there is less chance of achieving length in the abdominals. The forward contraction has the effect of squashing the abdominals. This makes them bulge upward rather than scoop. The exercise then becomes strained and ineffective.

With the knee joint at a right angle (feet farther away from the bottom), performance can improve, with increased effect on the muscle worked, as long as the abdominals are scooped in. With the knee joint at greater than a right angle (obtuse angle), the hip flexors are more elongated, and, if the lower back remains flat on the floor and the person is in a B-Line, the exercise is more challenging. If the pull of the hip flexors of the thigh is further reduced, the abdominals will work more effectively (see Exercise 25 with cushion under the knees).

Strength in length would be the epitome of muscle tone for almost every athlete. Female classical ballet dancers find that they are extremely flexible but not strong enough in their extreme ranges of movement. To them this is a weakness. But however desirable the strength factor is to them, most ballet dancers would not be caught dead in a weight training gym, for fear their muscles would become too bulky!

On the other hand, triathletes would welcome more flexibility without compromising their strength. But most of them would never be caught dead in a ballet class! Pilates' techniques can cater to both groups. Dancers can, with the correct use of weights, gain greater strength without fear of bulking their muscles. Triathletes can improve their flexibility without compromising their strength or speed. In fact, both could benefit from one common factor: the reduced risk of injury.

Elongation during the entire movement, through the full range of movement and during all repetitions, requires concentration and effort. As the muscle tires, the first thing to happen is the reduction in the lengthening of the muscle. This happens because the muscle can work more easily in a more contracted position. When you find that you cannot maintain your muscle elongation, stop the exercise. Continue only when you are able to maintain an elongated line.

6. Questions

Once the preceding five principles of the formula have been systematically performed, in the space of five seconds, the final and most important part of the equation remains: a checklist of all of the above, and more. Even when you have mentally assessed and corrected each movement, you might not be performing the exercise correctly. There are several ways to assess this. The following question can help you to correct the movement by returning to the formula:

Where do you feel the exercise working, and at what level on the work scale or stretch scale (whichever applies to the exercise)?

You should feel the exercise working in the muscle groups intended for that movement alone. For example, when you exercise the legs or lower limbs, the shoulders should not be hunching or straining. A simpler way of visualizing the movement of the limb is to concentrate on the movement of the bone itself and not the muscle. This way, you may be able to gain better control without straining.

There are many areas where things can go wrong. The rule is, If it feels uncomfortable or hurts, don't do it!

Common sense should dictate your actions at all times. Some of the most important areas to focus on are listed in the following section. This is by no means an exhaustive list, but as a guide, it can introduce an understanding of correct and safe muscle movement. This can give you a greater sense of awareness of the moving body

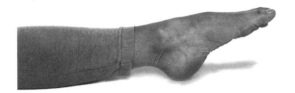

Figure 26(a). Softly pointed feet

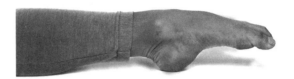

Figure 26(b). In the pointed position
(plantar flexion)

and encourage you to listen to your body when it talks to you.

BODY AWARENESS AND POSTURE

Getting to know your body is an important start to your Pilates program or, indeed, to any exercise program. As people develop physically, they also develop physical habits. Some of these may have taken years to develop, such as lifting objects in a certain way. Whatever the reason, when performing any task our bodies prefer to move along the path of least resistance. That path is accommodated by our subconscious. It is stored in our memory banks for future reference when we make the same, or similar, movements. Our bodies will automatically want to cheat on us when we perform many of life's everyday movements.

Many of these movements may be incorrect, such as walking with the arches of our feet dropped (pronated). This may explain why some people get headaches and others get lower back pain. However, most of us are not aware that such a movement could be the cause of our symptoms. Understanding and correcting the body's smallest imbalances or incorrect positioning can eliminate many of the minor, or major, aches and pains we become so accustomed to living with.

By becoming more aware of your body, and of the space within which it moves, you can gain greater understanding of your physical being. Mentally identifying and feeling individual parts of your body without having to move those parts may be difficult at first. However, when you achieve this, you can more easily understand how to move correctly. The result is that your physical and mental reflexes become more heightened; you can judge distances better, control the amount of effort you apply to physical tasks, and even relieve physical stress and mental anxiety.

Understanding your body also means listen-

ing to it when it reacts adversely to situations. It means not pushing it when you think you can perform a task but you realize that physically you have even slight doubts. As you develop your body with this program, you will begin to realize that without correct mental focus, your movements become sloppy and ineffective. Mentally, you also feel the same. It is important to realize that when your body has performed several repetitions of a movement as correctly as possible, and the extra one is not up to standard, then you should not continue with the remaining repetitions. One perfectly executed movement is worth any number of sloppy ones!

There are several key phrases that you will come across often in this book. They are essential to the basic control of the exercise and the achievement of beneficial results.

When you think you have gone as far as you can, extend it!

When moving the limbs or any part of the body, you can gain a greater feeling of working all muscles, especially the unused, smaller ones, by lengthening through the movement. For example, when standing or lying on your back, maintain a B-Line and keep the ribs lengthened away from the hips, while also pressing the shoulder blades to the hips. This requires more abdominal contraction and helps to keep the spine long and more flexible, as well as alleviating pressure on the vertebrae and discs.

When working on lengthening the arms or legs, do not lock the knee or elbow joints. This can cause stress on those joints. If these joints are hyperextended, then the bones are merely being locked together and the muscles will strain rather than work. You should also avoid too much of a bend, because that will not allow the muscle to lengthen and will restrict mobility of the limb from the socket. With the joint unlocked it is still

possible to lengthen out of the socket (without moving the hip or shoulder) to attain the mobility required.

ESTABLISHING CORRECT POSTURE

Foot Positions

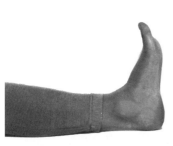

**Figure 27.
Inverted (sickle) feet**

The feet are an integral part of any exercise. Not to be regarded just as attachments at the end of our legs, the feet are continuously working. At no time should they be flopping around and left unattended.

When standing, imagine that each of your feet is like a tripod (see "The Tripod Position," p. 32). When you maintain this equal loading while moving the rest of the body, you will feel as if you were anchored to the floor. In this way, you can achieve a key element of good posture. Work the abdominals as described below, keeping the legs straight but not locked. Lift the ribs from the hips in a vertical line, maintain the B-Line, relax the shoulders to the hips, and lengthen the neck.

In the pointed position (Figure 26(b)), the feet are pointed with the joint between the big toe and the second toe in line with the center of the kneecap. This line of strength prevents the foot from either inversion (turning in) or eversion (turning out). The stretch should be felt on the top of the foot, and you should feel a lengthening sensation rather than a cramped pointing of the toes. Attempting to overstretch through the toes can result in a cramping of the arches of the feet. If this occurs, softly point the feet (Figure 26(a)).

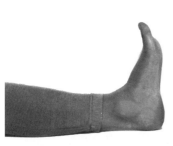

**Figure 28. Flexed position
(dorsi flexion)**

To achieve the flexed position, or dorsi flexion (Figure 28), press through the heels as far as possible. This should draw the toes toward your knees without curling them back. If the toes do tend to curl back, draw the balls of your feet toward you. This may take some practice. If, when you flex the feet, the calves feel excessively tight, stretch them before continuing with the rest of the program.

In Figures 29(a) and (b), the feet are shown both flexed and turned out, and pointed and turned out. When turning out, imagine the muscles of the inner thigh doing the work, rather than forcing the rotation from the knees or the feet.

Toning

Most women would like to tone the following muscle areas:

- The back of the arms.

- The section of abdominals below the navel.

- The buttocks.

- The outside of the hips.

- The back of the thighs.

Most men are principally interested in toning the entire abdominal area.

If we could keep the muscles toned continually, fatty deposits would have less chance of accumulating in these areas. For example, how often do we find fatty deposits on the front of the thighs? Because we are continuously walking, climbing stairs, jogging, or running, the quadriceps muscles rarely have a chance to rest in our

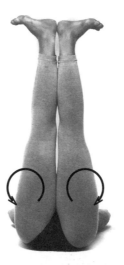 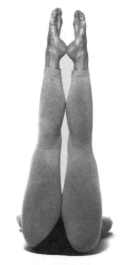 

**Figure 29(a).
Legs extended, feet
flexed and turned out**

**Figure 29(b).
Legs extended, feet
pointed and turned out**

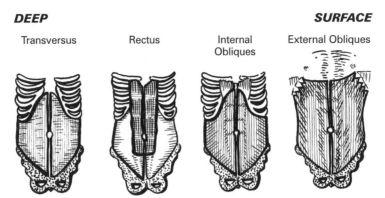

DEEP			SURFACE
Transversus	Rectus	Internal Obliques	External Obliques

Figure 30. Abdominal muscles

everyday routines. We do not have to worry about toning this group.

On the other hand, the buttocks are not often continually held firm in our normal, daily routines. Hence, the muscles there become slack and require extra work to reshape them to the desired size or shape. Squeezing the buttocks is not essential to maintaining good tone and may, ultimately, produce more bulk. When standing, keeping the buttocks pinched is preferable.

To firm this muscle group (the gluteus maximus), sit in a chair and imagine that you are holding a coin just inside the cheeks of the buttocks. Stand up out of the chair without dropping the coin, and keep the buttocks pinched. Do you notice how, automatically, the gluteals want to release, and all the effort transfers to the quadriceps? It may take some practice to learn to hold the gluteals on a regular basis. Perform this pinching of the buttocks whenever you are standing or sitting. This will reduce the need to use heavy, unnecessary exercise routines that can build bulk and create tighter lower back muscles.

The Center

The abdominals provide support for the back in its function of keeping the body erect. They also assist in the rotation of the torso.

This is easily shown by the following: Allow your stomach muscles to go slack. Notice what happens to your posture: You begin to slump. The shoulders move forward and down and the body becomes shorter. This can also lead to reduced breathing capacity as the lungs become squashed. Now sit upright on your sit bones without arching the back. (Sit as upright as possible without arching the back. Can you feel the two bones in your bottom that you are sitting on? These are known as the "sit bones.") Notice that at once your stomach pulls in toward your spine. The lower back muscles also engage to straighten the back. In addition, this has the effect of not only making you sit taller but also supporting the back and lifting pressure off of it.

Another way of illustrating this is to sit as though you were lifting your ribs vertically away from your hips, without allowing your ribs to move forward or the shoulders to hunch. If everyone were to keep such length between the ribs and the hips and maintain the B-Line, I am certain that up to 30 percent of all back problems could be more easily solved. This positioning of the spine is similar to alleviating the pressure on the vertebrae and discs by separating them from each other. This, in turn, can take some of the pressure off any nerves that are being impinged. If this

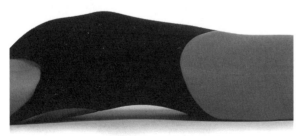

Figure 31(a).

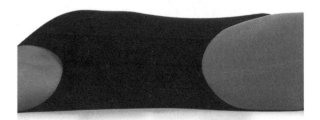

Figure 31(b).

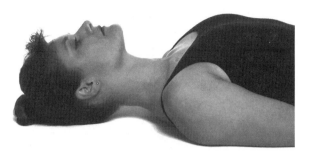

Figure 32(a). Do not allow the neck to arch

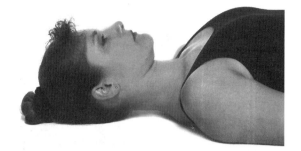

Figure 32(b). Lengthen the back of the neck

position can be maintained while the body is in motion, not only will the posture improve but mobility in the spine will increase.

Supine Position: Lying on Your Back

Place a mat on the floor and lie down on your back, feet extended and together and hands relaxed by your sides. You will observe that there is an arch in the lower back (Figure 31(a)). If this position is too uncomfortable, bend both legs very slightly. Place your hand in the space between your back and the floor and put your body in the B-Line. Can you feel the abdominal muscles engaging? (Do not push your feet on the floor or tilt your pelvis up to the ceiling.) By putting your body in the B-Line, you also engage the mid- and upper abdominal sections.

Remove the hand and continue to maintain the B-Line. Can you feel how much more deeply you are now working from the abdominal area? You may even feel as if the back itself were pressing to the floor (Figure 31(b)). This is one method of identifying and feeling your "center." It is the area from which all controlled strength and flowing movement emanate.

It is a common error to feel that if the back is not flat on the floor, then the back is not flat. The attempt here is to keep the back supported while the spine is in a normal, or neutral, position, one in which the hips are neither tilted in a tuck nor extended to arch the back.

Neck

When lying on your back, do not allow the neck to arch, as this will tighten the neck muscles and jut the chin forward. Lengthen the back of the neck to stretch these muscles and improve thoracic/cervical postural muscles.

Tension in the neck (and shoulders) can lead to poor posture and severe headaches. Tight trapezius and cervical muscles make the chin jut forward and create an arch in the neck. To create positive muscle control, press the shoulders to the floor and slowly draw the tip of the chin slightly down toward the rib cage while lengthening the crown of the head to the ceiling. Can you feel the stretch in the back of the neck? This feeling may even extend down the upper back toward the shoulder blades. Do not squash the chin to the chest.

Sitting

In a sitting position, most people have the tendency to slump (Figure 33(b)). When sitting, lift up out of the hips or sit tall on your sit bones. Imagine your spine is similar to a rod. This rod is perfectly upright, perpendicular to the floor, running from the base of your spine through the crown of your head. Now imagine that your torso is sliding up that rod, while your hips remain anchored to the ground, your body is in the B-Line, and your shoulders are relaxed to the floor (Figure 33(a)).

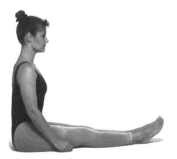

Figure 33(a). In a sitting position, perfectly upright

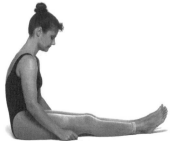

Figure 33(b). Incorrect sitting position

Shoulders

Neck and shoulder tension is a common problem for most people, whether they exercise or not. This tension is caused by the trapezius muscles. Often when we are encountered with a sudden shock or surprise, our arms, shoulders, and neck immediately tense in an almost defensive reaction. When we lift objects, even when we hold a baby on the hip, we hunch the shoulders. Then, when our friends give us a neck or shoulder rub, they comment on how these muscles are "as hard as rocks."

This tension can be caused by situations as various as sitting in front of a typewriter or computer all day, or worrying about the results of an

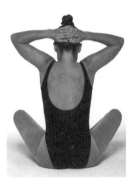 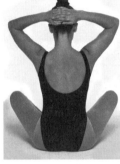

Figure 34(a).
Incorrect

Figure 34(b).
Correct

exam! Tension shortens the muscle group, as tension does with any muscles, which hunches (and slightly rounds) the shoulders and arches the neck. To reverse this process, sit in an upright position and start by feeling the tension in the neck and shoulder muscles with your fingers. While gently applying pressure to the shoulder muscles, hunch your shoulders. Now, gently allow the shoulders to release by pressing the shoulder blades to the floor as hard as you can while growing your spine to the ceiling. At the same time, slightly squeeze the shoulder blades together. This has the effect of opening the chest and allowing a slight release of the pectoral muscles that round the shoulders forward. It may even cause some discomfort between the shoulder blades as the muscles stretch. Repeat this movement several times, and feel the tension release further each time.

Another method of feeling the tension release is to place your hands on the top of your head, with your elbows forward. (If you place your el-

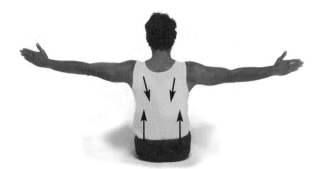

Figure 35.
Press shoulder blades to floor,
lift ribs from hips

bows wide open, the trapezius muscle remains in a contracted position.) Sit with your arms extended away from the body at shoulder height, lengthening through your fingertips.

Your neck and shoulders may already feel tense. Hunch them up as much as you can. Do you notice that the chin also tends to jut forward?

Now focus on the following:

1. Press the shoulder blades to the floor as hard as you can, with a deep sigh out.

2. Lengthen farther through the fingertips.

3. Grow as tall as you can out of your hips.

4. Slightly squeeze the shoulder blades together without creating further tension in the back.

Repeat the movement by hunching only 10 percent as much as before. Now perform the release procedure above and hold it for twenty seconds while breathing normally. Repeat four more times and then rest your hands by your sides. Do you feel taller? More relaxed? Does your body feel lighter? Do you feel more relaxed mentally? By contracting the muscles opposite to the ones that automatically create the tension, you can use positive muscle control to negate the effects of not only physical but also mental tension.

Imprinting

Because the spine is a major focal point of movement for the rest of the body, it is important to keep it supple and strong. The movement of the spine when you get up off the floor or lie down should resemble that of leaving an imprint of the spine in soft sand. When you lower or raise the

torso to or from the floor, each vertebra should be moved one at a time, without any sharp or jerky movements. Some analogies may help you to achieve this:

NOTES

1. Imagine the spine is like a string of pearls being lowered (or raised) one at a time.

2. Imagine that your spine is stuck to a wheel; as the wheel smoothly turns, so does each vertebra move one at a time.

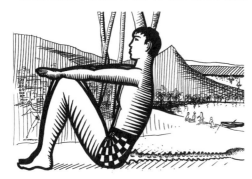

Figure 36. Imprinting

In a sitting position when curling the spine up or down, you can gain more flexibility in the back by reaching forward through the fingertips while rounding the back.

CHAPTER 4

Making Your Pilates
Workout Effective and Safe

There are only three

things in life that will

help us to live longer.

Strength and suppleness

together—and a good

sense of humor.

ANONYMOUS

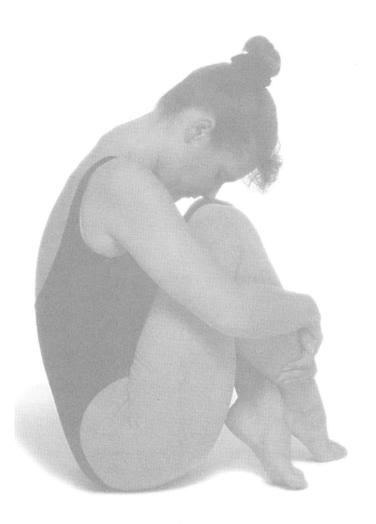

Although we are promoting isolation of muscles to attain a leaner, longer body with control and precision of movement, we should keep in mind that the body works as a whole. Even when you attempt to isolate a particular muscle for a stretch, other muscles may come into play. It is true that the toe bone is connected to the cheek bone via a complex arrangement of tissue, muscles, connecting joints, and mental perception.

WARM-UP AND STRETCHING BEFORE YOUR WORKOUT

Stretching is an all-important part of warming up the muscles before any physical activity. It "wakes up" the muscles by providing an infusion of blood and nutrients into the more open tissue. This makes the muscles more pliable and flexible, and the underlying joints are also able to move more freely.

There are two main types of stretches: dynamic (involving motion) and static (involving no motion).

The following sensible stretching practices should be followed when performing stretches:

1. Stretch the muscle gradually.

2. If you feel any joint pain, reduce the pressure on the joint by doing either (a) or (b) (see below). If you still feel joint pain, do not continue.

CASE STUDY

While attempting a normal hamstring stretch, keeping the back in an upright position and holding onto the bench, the patient felt a cramping of the muscles in the middle back area just below the shoulder blades. The cause of this was that, when the patient attempted to increase the forward lean and, thereby, increase the stretch for the hamstring, the latissimus dorsi and lower trapezium gripped. The client was also found to be tightening the muscles between the shoulder blades (the rhomboids). This was easily corrected by depressing the shoulders and slightly rounding the upper back. The pain disappeared, and the effectiveness of the hamstring stretch was maintained.

a) Reduce the angle at the joint. For example, when you do a seated hamstring stretch, if you feel more pain behind the knee joint than in the hamstring, bend the knee until you feel more of a hamstring stretch.

b) Control the rotation of the joint. For example, if you perform side splits and feel pressure in the knee joint, this may be because the femur is internally rotated. Externally rotate the thigh until you feel only the adductor.

3. Do not stretch injured or torn muscles.

4. If you have achieved maximum range of movement and do not feel the stretch, continue the movement as a means of mobilizing the joint and loosening up before working the muscle.

5. If stretching a group of muscles affects another group (e.g., a thoracic stretch strains the shoulder joint), do not continue without further guidance.

6. After the muscle has been worked, stretch all muscle groups. This is important in order to

a) Reduce bulking of the muscle.

b) Reduce the risk of injury to joints, muscles, and tendons.

c) Reduce post-exercise soreness in the muscle.

d) Maintain and increase joint mobility.

e) Increase flexibility.

f) Help you to cool down.

When starting any exercise routine, it is necessary to limber up before launching into the meat of the program. This can generally take the form of a five-minute bike ride, a jog around the block, or *effective stretching* that gradually lengthens and mobilizes the muscle groups for longer than ninety seconds at a time.

Gentle stretching can also form a part of this warm-up for those incapable of engaging in these methods of warming up, those who find these

methods uncomfortable, or those with injuries. Stretching and strengthening the uninjured muscle groups, by isolating them, is an ideal means of staying in shape for those with any injury. As long as there are no effects on the injured muscles, tendons, joints, or ligaments, or the area immediately surrounding the injury, exercising the uninjured muscles can keep the body toned and functioning and is much better than not exercising at all.

For the average person, substituting this extended stretching for a warm-up routine is not detrimental. In fact, in some cases it is more beneficial and safer than other warm-up routines.

If the weather is cold, or if your muscles feel excessively tight, then you should spend extra time on stretching. The time of day when you should stretch is entirely up to you. Some people feel much better stretching in the early morning (to wake themselves up), while others feel as if they are unable to move at all until the end of the working day, when the body has been mobilized and feels looser.

There is no evidence to suggest that practicing extended stretching techniques is detrimental to physical achievement when performing a controlled, nonstrenuous exercise program. In fact, most people using Pilates' techniques report that they feel more energized, more flexible, and less mentally and physically stressed at the end of their stretching routines.

In order for the muscle to achieve its maximum range of movement, a continual stretch into the specific muscle area is required. Combined with the correct breathing technique (in through the nose for five seconds, followed with a sigh out through the mouth for five seconds without depressing the chest), stretching helps to increase blood flow to the muscles. This helps a great deal in improving the elasticity of the muscle as well as in the elimination of lactic acid from the muscle group.

The Start Stretches (Exercises 3–6a) described at the beginning of the program are intended to stretch isolated muscle groups. The ideal order for stretching is to start with the back (lower and upper) and shoulders, continue with the hamstrings, and then move on to the thighs. Because some muscle groups are interdependent, stretching some muscles may reduce the need to stretch others. For example, stretching tight calves may reduce the need to stretch the hamstrings. Therefore, after stretching the back and shoulders, it would be prudent to stretch the calves before continuing with a hamstring stretch.

POINTERS FOR SAFE EXERCISING

1. If at any time a stretch or exercise feels uncomfortable or painful, reduce its intensity by reducing the range of movement or easing the pressure on the joint.

2. If you feel sharp pain or pain in another part of the body, stop the exercise. Seek the advice of a qualified instructor on the movements you are doing.

3. If a movement feels too easy, first follow the principles and formula to enhance the quality of the movement, then increase the intensity of the exercise by progressing to the next version of the movement.

4. If you ever feel your neck straining during a supine exercise, support it with cushions or pillows. The exercise may then be completed without any strain on the breathing or on muscles that are not the working ones.

5. Whenever performing an exercise that requires you to be on your back, maintain the B-Line and flatten the back (without tilting the pelvis), unless otherwise stated in the instructions. If, as the exercise progresses, you feel that your back is arching, it may mean one of several things:

   a) Your legs may be too far away from the center. Draw the knees closer to the chest or bring the legs more vertically into the air.

   b) If the position requires the head and shoulders to be contracted forward (shoulder blades just off the floor, ribs and hips in the same plane), this contraction may slowly be releasing as the exercise progresses. Attempt to maintain the contraction at all times.

   c) The abdominal muscles may be gradu-

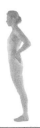

ally weakening, and the back muscles may be beginning to take over. If the back comes off the floor even one millimeter (if you can slide a ruler between your back and the floor), then the back may be doing more work than the abdominals. Stop the exercise. There is no point in continuing the exercise if the powerhouses of the anatomy, the abdominals, are no longer controlling the movement.

6. Challenge yourself! Progress can be achieved only by increasing the intensity or range of movement of the exercise by a small percentage each time. Follow the program as closely as you can, and you will gain more confidence and body awareness. You will feel like a different person!

THE STRUCTURE OF THE EXERCISE PROGRAM

1. Prerequisite Exercises

In order to perform certain intermediate or advanced exercises comfortably and safely, it is necessary to first do some basic muscle strengthening or stretching. These prerequisite exercises will be described at the beginning of the exercise section.

2. Purpose of the Exercise / Muscles Worked

Each exercise will have a section describing the muscles that are to be worked and the purpose of the exercise. In many instances there will also be an explanation of how the exercise relates to a "non-exercise" movement. This is where we can see the use of what is being achieved in the routine and how those muscles need to function outside an exercise situation.

3. Description of the Exercise and Correct Breathing

The description of the exercise includes the following:

■ Starting position

■ Back position

■ Breathing

■ Exercise

4. Key Points

There are major mental or physical points to consider when doing any movement. Slight movements, though possibly minor, can produce a considerable difference in the effectiveness of the exercise. Remember, even a centimeter's deviation in the placement of your body can mean up to 50 percent difference in the effectiveness of the exercise!

5. Care

At the end of the description of each exercise are care notes. These notes discuss the most commonly encountered problems that may arise during the movement and how to counteract these stresses safely. They should answer most major questions that might come up about the exercise.

6. Repetitions

For each exercise, I suggest the ideal number of sets and repetitions. Remember, at the end of each repetition it is important to go on to the following repetition without resting in between, because if you rest the muscle will relax and need to be reconnected for the next repetition. One movement should flow into the next. At all times you should maintain muscle tone and muscle identification through isolation, as well as continuing to breathe deeply. Thus, you can improve your mental and physical stamina and endurance, which will increase your confidence in what your body can achieve.

Complete only the number of repetitions with which you are comfortable. If you can manage only six repetitions before you start to feel that the exercise is not working properly or effectively, then stop after six. In this case, add one repetition each week until you have reached the required number. I have used the example of six repetitions because this is more than 50 percent of the generally required amount. By completing more than 50 percent, you will be closer to finishing and will have passed the psychological halfway barrier.

PILATES' EXERCISE ROUTINES

The programs that follow have been designed with careful thought to the differing abilities of the individuals undertaking the routines. If any of the exercises are too difficult, please follow the instructions under "Pointers for Safe Exercising."

Each program is slightly more challenging than the last. If you feel that any exercise from one section is too difficult, substitute an exercise from a previous section without a drastic overhaul of the entire section. You may tailor your program to your own needs and abilities until you are able to follow the routines suggested. The following are the routines presented here:

1. *The Warm-Up.* For loosening the tight major muscles of the legs, lower back, and shoulders.

2. *The Routine for Lower Back Pain and Weak Abdominals.* For those who have minor lower back pain that does not involve referred pain (down the legs, etc.), and for those with weak abdominals.

3. *The Basic Routine.* For those starting an exercise program.

4. *The Intermediate Routine.* For those who have no back pain and are of a reasonable-to-average fitness level.

5. *The Advanced Routine.* For those who can complete the Intermediate Routine with ease, exercise regularly, and require a challenge.

6. *More Advanced Exercises.* For those who need a greater challenge than the advanced program.

7. *Theraband Exercises.* For gaining strength with resistance.

Remember to seek medical approval or advice from a qualified Pilates practitioner before embarking on any exercise program, especially if you have never attempted these exercises before.

I apologize, in advance, for the length of the explanations in some of the exercises. If, at first, you cannot understand them all to make full use of them, do not worry. Start with only two or three of the instructions for each exercise. As you become familiar and comfortable with these, then add another instruction. I feel it is better to give you as much information as possible, so that it will be available when you are ready to make use of all of it. This not only provides you with the most comprehensive set of instructions ever written for Pilates' exercises but should also answer all your questions in relation to the exercises.

You should wear snug but comfortable clothing. If possible, place a mirror where you can see yourself in order to correct any postural deviations that you would not otherwise notice. It would be ideal to have a friend read the instructions to you, once you have a mental picture of what the exercise looks like from the photos or diagrams. For all the floor routines, use a thick but firm mat to lie on.

When embarking on the program, try to commit yourself to it for at least three times a week for six to eight weeks. The first two weeks will be the toughest. Any good, effective exercise program takes time to establish itself within your muscle memory. It took years to create the body you now have—it is not going to change overnight. Stick to it, and you will gradually start to see changes. You will be glad you persevered. Good luck!

P.S. I have included a "Notes" section for you at the end of most of the exercises. Use this area to take notes on ideas that you may have for future reference.

At the end of the exercise section, I have included suggested programs for daily routines from the four sections. Each week, add an extra exercise from the section, until you are able to complete all the exercises comfortably. Then move on to the next section.

CHAPTER 5

The Warm-Up

Not only is health

a normal condition,

but it is a duty not

only to attain but

to maintain it.

J. PILATES

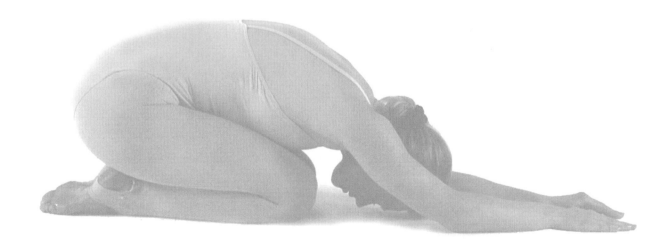

Exercise 1
RESTING POSITION

REPETITIONS: One set of ten breaths in and ten breaths out.

BREATHING: Breathe in and out deeply and slowly for ten breaths.

PREREQUISITE: This position can be used at any time during the program.

PURPOSE: To relax and allow the spine to stretch.

EXERCISE DESCRIPTION:

Starting Position: Kneel back on your haunches, with your toes extended.

    a) Keeping your buttocks on the heels as much as possible, slowly breathe out and curl the spine forward while sliding your fingers on the floor ahead of you.

    b) Stretch all the way forward through your fingertips, while pressing your shoulder blades to your hips. Rest your forehead on the floor. Breathe in without moving.

    c) Relax in this position.

KEY POINTS: On every breath out, press the buttocks onto your heels and lengthen your chest to your knees. This is a very small movement. When you feel you have lengthened as far as you can, relax in this position. After several breaths, attempt a further small lengthening movement.

CARE: If you feel any discomfort in the knees, place a cushion behind the knees. This will keep the buttocks off the heels and will allow for a more comfortable stretch.

NOTES

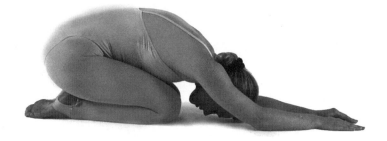

Exercise 2
STANDING SPINE ROLL

PREREQUISITE: This is a basic prerequisite for all exercises.

PURPOSE: To loosen up the spine, hamstrings, and lower back.

EXERCISE DESCRIPTION:

Starting Position: Stand as tall as you can with your feet shoulder-distance apart and parallel. Imagine your spine is stuck to a wall. Do the B-Line, pelvis slightly tucked under (posterior tilt), shoulders relaxed.

  a) Bend your knees slightly and breathe out deeply as you slowly and sequentially peel your vertebrae off the wall one at a time: lower your chin forward to your rib cage, then ribs to hips, while pressing your lower back into the imaginary wall.

  b) Halfway down, take a deep breath in, and then with a deep breath out, relax the body as far as it will comfortably go, keeping the knees bent. If you cannot touch your toes, do not force yourself to do so. At the bottom of the movement, take a deep breath into the chest, maintaining the B-Line.

  c) Breathe out and return to the standing position by reversing the movement, imprinting your spine onto the imaginary wall, or imagine stacking your vertebrae one on top of the other. Start the movement by tucking the pelvis and drawing the hips to the rib cage, engage the lower abdominals, then press the middle and upper abdominals to the spinal wall. This movement should be felt in the anterior portion of the body (the abdominals).

KEY POINTS: Keep the body weight over the feet, which should be in the tripod position. Lengthen the ribs from the hips on the upward roll. Flatten the stomach, relax the shoulders.

CARE: If you feel the slightest back strain on the upward roll, bend the knees until only the abdominals are doing the work. Do not force yourself to touch your toes if you are unable to do so comfortably.

REPETITIONS: One set of ten.

BREATHING: Breathe out on the way down, breathe in at the point of flexion (relaxation), and breathe out on the way up.

ADVANCED: Straighten the legs a bit more each time you do the movement.

NOTES

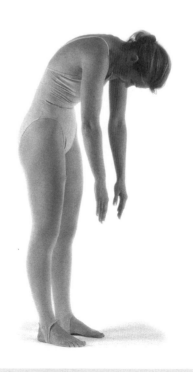

PREREQUISITE: This is a basic prerequisite exercise for the whole program.

PURPOSE: To stretch the lower and middle back, and to open the groin area.

EXERCISE DESCRIPTION:

Starting Position: Sit upright on the sit bones as if against a wall, with knees drawn toward the groin and dropped open, soles of the feet together. Ensure that the lower 6 inches at the base of the back is perfectly erect at all times. If it is not, place the feet farther away from the groin or sit up against a wall and allow the spine to touch it without leaning against it at any time. The body should not be slumped into the hips. Sit as tall on the sit bones as possible.

a) Reach the arms to the ceiling, stretching the spine; bend the elbows and place the fingers down the back between the shoulder blades. Imagine that you have suction cups on your finger tips, so as you curl forward the hands do not slide up toward the neck. This will increase the intensity of the stretch. Keep the shoulders relaxed when lifting the ribs from the hips.

b) Breathe out as you curl the head forward onto the chest and down toward the rib cage, letting the upper spine follow. You are attempting to roll your nose toward your B-Line, keeping the lower 6 inches of the spine as upright as possible. Let the chest rise and fall with the breathing. If this is difficult because of the compression of the chest in this position, breathe into the back (See "Breathing," pp. 22–25). Press the knees open to the floor.

c) Hold the position for the breath in, without moving, then curl further forward toward the B-Line on the next breath out. Curl as far into the B-Line as possible on the first movement. After this the movements are very small, if at all.

This movement is very slight and can be felt quite strongly in the muscles on either side of the spine, in the lower back, or across the shoulder blades.

KEY POINTS: The lumbar spine should be perpendicular. Lift out of the hips without hunching the shoulders. Maintain the B-Line, elbows close to and behind the ears. Relax the shoulders and neck, curve from the rib cage. Sit tall on the sit bones at all times. Press the knees open to the floor to open the groin. If this is uncomfortable, keep the knees relaxed open. If the feet are too close to the groin, you may feel as if you were rolling back onto the hips. Place the feet farther away from the body until you are sitting tall comfortably (unsupported by the hands). Do not allow the body to lean forward so the head moves over the feet. This means a lean from the hips rather than a bend at the rib cage, changing the muscles required to be stretched. On the breath in, do not allow the body to move at all. Do not cross the hands to avoid any strain on the neck when contracting forward.

CARE: If you feel the shoulders hunch or the neck strain, relax the shoulders. Keep the shoulder blades in line with the hips. Do not force the chin onto the chest: instead, roll it comfortably down to the rib cage, and then nose to the B-Line.

REPETITIONS: One set of ten breaths in and ten out.

BREATHING: Breathe in while allowing the chest to expand through all areas, especially the sides and back. If breathing is difficult, breathe "into the back" or do not contract forward too far.

VARIATIONS: Sit tall on your sit bones, and maintain the B-Line. Repeat the exercise as above, moving the feet to the different positions described below for the ten-breath repetition.

DURATION: Ten slow breaths in and out, contracting farther forward on the breath out.

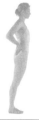

Exercise 4

Position your legs straight and together in front, feet pointed. Make sure your knees are pointing up to the ceiling so the thighs are not turned out. Press the ankle bones together. If the feeling is too strong behind the knees, bend the knees only slightly.

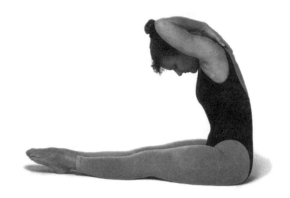

Exercise 5

Place your legs straight and together in front, feet flexed and pressing through the heels. This should be felt comfortably in the spine and mildly to strongly in the hamstrings.

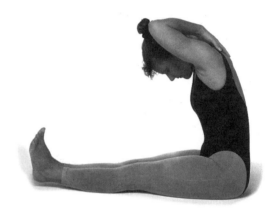

Exercise 6

Place the left leg straight in front of the left hip, foot flexed, right leg bent at the knee with the sole of the foot against the inside of the left knee of the extended leg. The hips should be square and the leg in line with the hip. Do not adjust the hips to establish the position—only adjust the legs.

Exercise 6a

Reverse legs as in Exercise 6.

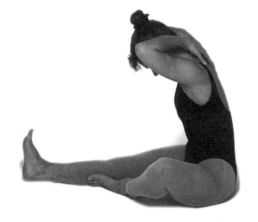

NOTES

Exercise 7
SPIRAL STRETCH

PREREQUISITE: To be able to correctly perform upper back stretches, with no problems or strain in the back whatsoever. Do not perform this stretch if you have any back problems or back pain.

PURPOSE: To stretch the sides between the armpit and the hips, lower back muscles, and shoulder joints.

EXERCISE DESCRIPTION:

Starting Position: Sit as in Exercise 6. Breathe in and reach both arms to the ceiling (left leg straight, right leg bent).

a) Put your body in the B-Line and rotate the torso to the right, rotating the center of the breastbone (sternum) past the point of the bent knee.

b) Breathe out and stretch the torso sideways along the extended leg. Hold onto the foot or the ankle of the straight leg with the left hand.

c) Breathe in without moving; while breathing out, bend the left elbow to try to lengthen the left armpit toward the left knee (without bending the knee). Stretch the right hand past the left foot and parallel to the floor. Breathe in, without moving. Repeat ten times.

d) To finish, lengthen both arms past the extended foot, reaching out of the hips to the ceiling (remaining rotated); then rotate back to the front position. Relax the hands by the sides. Change sides.

KEY POINTS: Keep the hips square, maintain the B-Line, and keep both sit bones on the floor. Lengthen through the spine, with the uppermost shoulder to the ceiling, and avoid overarching in the lower back. Try to maintain the top arm/elbow behind the top ear. The more rotation you can achieve, the better the stretch.

CARE: If the rotation feels uncomfortable in any part of the body, stop. Keep the body directly over the extended leg and slightly in front of it for a better stretch.

REPETITIONS: Breathe in ten times and breathe out ten times. Do one set on each side.

BREATHING: Breathe in as you hold the position; breathe out as you stretch over the extended leg.

VARIATIONS: If you are flexible enough to hold the foot of the extended leg with the top hand, do so. Place the other hand on the floor inside the extended leg. When breathing out, bend the elbow of the top hand to the ceiling, holding onto the foot for leverage, and walk the fingers of the bottom hand along the floor to stretch that side. On every breath out, rotate and lengthen the torso further. Press the hips of the bent leg into the floor for a better stretch. Maintain the B-line, especially on the breath in.

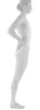

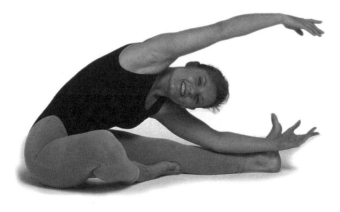

Exercise 8-1
CALF STRETCHES

PREREQUISITE: None.

PURPOSE: To stretch and strengthen the calf muscles (gastrocnemius and soleus).

EXERCISE DESCRIPTION:

Starting Position: Stand with the balls of the feet on the edge of a step. Place a tennis ball between the ankles to prevent the feet from rolling outward on the rise. Place a thick pad between the knees to prevent them from rolling in and to help to connect the inner thigh muscles.

   a) Put your body in the B-Line with a slight tuck of the pelvis. Breathe in and rise up onto the balls of the feet as high as possible. Do not drop the tennis ball.

Think of working the muscles in the feet rather than working from the calves.

   b) Breathe out as the feet lower to below the level of the step, pressing the heels down as far as possible. As the heels lower below the horizontal level, squeeze the pad and lightly turn out the upper thighs. The knees and upper thighs have a tendency to roll in at this point.

KEY POINTS: Do not drop the ball or the pad. If the knees are too far apart, use a thicker pad. The point of the rise should be on the ball of the foot between the big toe and the second toe. This should be in alignment with the center of the kneecap.

CARE: Do not allow the lower back to arch at any time. Tuck, if required, to prevent this. Do not drop into the heels; lower and press down gradually.

REPETITIONS: Fifteen to twenty repetitions.

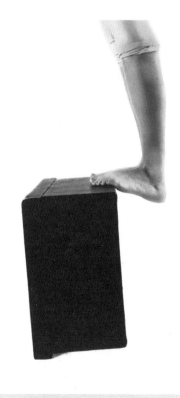

Exercise 8-2
ALTERNATING CALF STRETCHES

PREREQUISITE: Exercise 8-1.

PURPOSE: To stretch the calves more than in the previous exercise, especially if one calf is tighter than the other.

EXERCISE DESCRIPTION:

Starting Position: Stand on the edge of a step on the balls of the feet. Get into the B-Line and, while breathing in, rise up onto the balls of the feet as high as possible. Imagine you are holding a tennis ball between the ankles.

  a) Breathe out as the right heel lowers below the level of the step, while the left leg stays high on the ball of the foot, bending the knee. Slightly turn out the right thigh to prevent the knee from rolling in.

  b) Breathe in as you rise up on the right foot only to the height of the left foot. Change feet and repeat with the left foot.

KEY POINTS: As in exercise 8-1. In addition, use the muscles of only one foot at a time. Do not let the hips swing out to the sides by sinking into them.

CARE: As in exercise 8-1.

REPETITIONS: Twenty repetitions, alternating legs.

VARIATION FOR THE SOLEUS: As the heel lowers below the horizontal position, bend the knee to stretch the soleus (the deeper layer of the calf muscles).

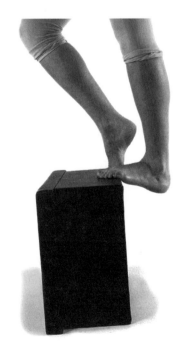

HAMSTRING STRETCH: BASIC

PREREQUISITE: This is a basic prerequisite exercise.

PURPOSE: To safely stretch the hamstring muscles for those with extremely tight hamstrings or with back pain.

EXERCISE DESCRIPTION:

Starting Position: Lie on your back with the knees bent at a right angle.

a) Bend one knee to the chest and place a long towel or Theraband around the heel.

b) Slowly extend the heel to the ceiling, while holding on to the towel. Keep extending the foot until you feel a strong stretch in the hamstring (not behind the knee). If the leg fully extends and there is no effect on the spine, move on to Exercise 9-2.

c) Breathe in, holding the position. Take a deep breath out and press the heel to the ceiling for more of a stretch, without the tailbone lifting off the mat.

KEY POINTS: Maintain the B-Line and keep the hips firmly pressed to the floor without arching the back. Place a cushion under the head if the neck arches. Do not hunch the shoulders or allow them to come off the mat.

CARE: Maintain the B-Line, and keep the shoulder blades slightly squeezed together and the neck long.

REPETITIONS: Ten breaths in and ten breaths out. Do two sets on each leg, alternating legs. It is important to alternate the legs rather than doing all twenty repetitions without stopping. This gives the muscle some breathing space before subjecting it to more stretching. By doing this you do not push the muscle to its limits without a break. Therefore, you get more benefit from the exercise, because you are able to do a better conscious stretch during the second set.

BREATHING: Breathe out as you press through the heel. Breathe in as you hold the position.

ADVANCED: As this exercise becomes easier, slowly straighten the bent leg. Continue to draw the leg being stretched toward the same shoulder, without bending the knee. As the stretched leg is able to maintain a straight position, gradually extend the leg on the mat to an almost straight position, without the back arching, foot flexed.

NOTES

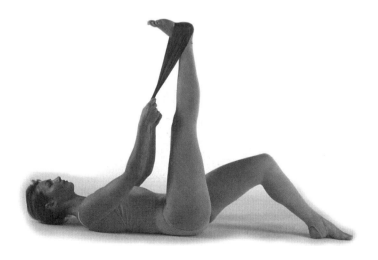

Exercise 9-2
HAMSTRING STRETCH 2

PREREQUISITE: Stretched calves.

PURPOSE: To perform a more specific stretch on the hamstring group.

EXERCISE DESCRIPTION:

Starting Position: Standing upright, place the right foot on a chair or table, with the leg extended up to hip level. If you are more flexible, you can raise the leg higher. Your left foot should be facing forward.

a) Keep the hips square and parallel, the foot flexed, and the kneecap pointed to the ceiling. Put your body in the B-line.

b) Keep the knee as straight as possible. Maintain the B-line and breathe out as you lean your chest forward. Imagine that on every breath out, you are growing taller as you lean forward out of the hips. Do not bend the head or chest to the knee. Keep the head upright at all times, stretching through the crown of the head to the ceiling.

c) Hold the position for the breath in; breathe out, lift, and lean forward farther (only a slight movement is required).

KEY POINTS: If you feel more pressure behind the knee than in the hamstring, bend the knee. Imagine someone is lifting you out of your lower back: lift up and away from the tailbone, almost as if you were attempting to arch the very lower part of the back. If performed correctly, this stretch should be immediate and quite strong. Keep the pelvis square and level to the floor. Keep the supporting leg firmly planted into the floor at all times directly below the hip. Flex the foot as much as possible to achieve more stretch. Maintain the B-line.

CARE: If you feel an uncomfortable stretch in any part of the back, do Exercise 8. If you feel tightness between the shoulder blades, round the shoulders slightly. If you feel a mild tightness in the lower back (from lifting out of the hips), bend very slightly from the lower back until the discomfort eases. Keep the hips square and level, keep the supporting leg directly under the hip, and be sure not to hyperextend the knee. Keep the upper back straight, leaning forward from the hip joint. If you feel too much pressure behind the knee, bend it. You should feel only the hamstring.

REPETITIONS: Breathe in and out ten times.

BREATHING: Breathe in as you lengthen the spine to the ceiling, and breathe out while opening the chest to the wall in front. Remain in this posture for ten breaths. On each out breath, extend farther up and forward to feel the stretch.

NOTES

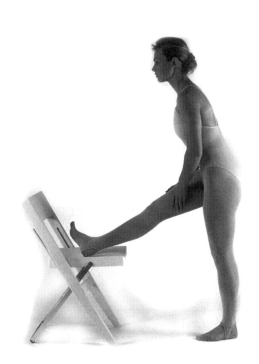

NOTES

a) Sit on one leg on a flat bench. In this position it is easier to keep the hips level. The leg on the ground is bent and the toe is facing forward. This is easier than the version above.

b) Standing (as in Exercise 9-2), raise the leg to a higher level than the hip. This action may begin to lift the hip, so use the hand of the same side to press the hip to the floor. This movement alone will create the start of the stretch.

c) Use the arms to lean the body farther forward by holding on to the leg or the bench and bending at the elbows.

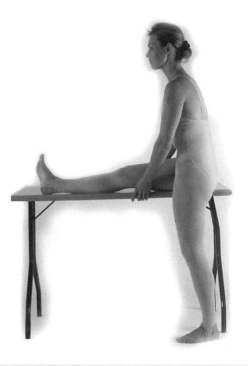

Exercise 11
THIGH STRETCH 1: PRONE

PREREQUISITE: This is a basic prerequisite exercise for those who cannot do Thigh Stretches 2 or 3.

PURPOSE: To stretch the thigh muscle group, especially for those with knee joint problems.

EXERCISE DESCRIPTION:

Starting Position: Lie face-down on a mat with a small, folded towel placed under the stomach to assist in maintaining the B-Line. Bend the right leg, drawing the foot to the buttock. Reach back with the right hand and grasp the foot. The body should remain in a straight line, without the shoulders twisting or the knee shifting away from a straight line with the hip. You should feel a mild to strong stretch along the front of the right thigh.

   a) Breathe out and bend the right elbow in order to bring the heel closer to the buttock, maintaining the B-Line and pressing the right hipbone to the floor. Hold the position for the breath in. Repeat ten times, drawing the heel closer to the buttock each time, while B-Lining to a greater extent. You should feel an extremely strong stretch in the middle of the thigh. Press the right hipbone into the floor.

KEY POINTS: The towel is meant to help prevent the back from arching and taking any pressure. If you are able to place the hipbone flat on the floor, then progress to Thigh Stretch 2, as long as you have no knee joint problems that may be triggered by putting pressure on one knee.

CARE: If you cannot bend the knee to the buttock comfortably, it is a clear indication that the thigh muscles are tight. If you feel any pressure in the back, it may be arching too much, or your body may not be in a straight line. Try placing a towel around the foot, hold on to the towel, and draw the foot toward the buttock. Make sure the foot is in a direct line with the buttock and drawn over to the inside of the thigh.

REPETITIONS: Two sets of ten breaths, alternating.

BREATHING: Ten breaths in and ten breaths out in each set.

NOTES

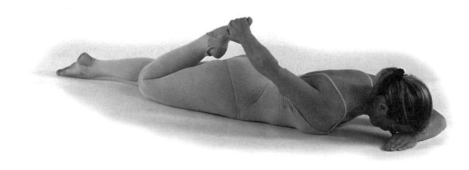

PREREQUISITE: This is a basic prerequisite exercise.

PURPOSE: To stretch the thighs and to connect the B-Line and open the lower back.

EXERCISE DESCRIPTION:

Starting Position: To stretch the left thigh, stand with the right leg on the floor and the left leg bent on a chair, or hold on to the left foot with the left hand. This requires some balance. Your balance will improve over time as you complete more stretches.

  a) Breathe out as you tuck the pelvis under. This can be greatly assisted by pressing the left buttock to the floor and drawing the pubic bone to the navel with the assistance of the right hand.

  b) Breathe in, and hold the position. Breathe out and tuck under more.

KEY POINTS: Remain leaning slightly forward all the time. This opens the lower back, and the continual tuck opens it even further.

Be sure that the hips are level and square before you start the exercise. The bent leg usually has a tendency to lift the hip on that side. By simply squaring the pelvis (parallel to the floor), you will feel a mild to strong stretch.

Ensure that the front of the thighs are level with each other. If the thigh being stretched is farther forward than the (other) supporting leg, press the knee down to the floor as much as possible while bringing it in line with the supporting leg, without arching the back. This should induce a stronger stretch with a small movement of the thigh downward.

CARE: You should feel this stretch very strongly on the quadriceps only (middle to top of the thigh) and no other place. (This pain level may exceed the nine level.) When the stretch stops, so should the pain. If the pain continues after the stretch has stopped, do not repeat. Sigh on the breath out, and relax the shoulders. The thigh stretch is the only one on which you may exceed the nine out of ten level. This is because the thigh muscle is an extremely tight muscle and can take the stretch. It is uncomfortable, but the discomfort ceases as soon as you stop the exercise. If it does not, stop doing the stretch.

REPETITIONS: Two sets of ten breaths in and ten breaths out, alternating legs.

BREATHING: Breathe in without moving; breathe out on the tuck.

NOTES

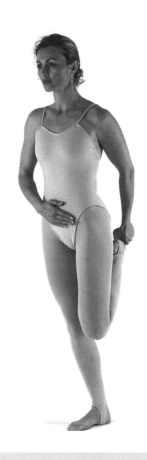

Exercise 13
THIGH STRETCH 3: KNEELING

PREREQUISITE: Achieving Thigh Stretch 2 without feeling much strain.

PURPOSE: To stretch the thigh muscles and iliopsoas, connect the B-Line, and open the lower back. (The iliopsoas is the muscle that attaches from the lower spine to the top of the thigh bone. If the abdominals are weak, this muscle tends to arch the lower back.)

EXERCISE DESCRIPTION:

Starting Position: To stretch the right thigh, place a thick towel or a piece of dense foam under the right knee, with the foot up against a wall or on a chair. If this is uncomfortable on the front of the foot, place a soft pad under the foot. This position is most easily achieved by placing the hands on the floor and then putting the knee/leg into position. Bend the left knee, place both hands on the left knee, and come into the upright position.

   a) The exercise now follows the same steps as Thigh Stretch 2.

   b) Place the right hand on the right buttock and the left hand just above the pubic bone. Press the buttock to the floor and draw the pubic bone to the navel.

KEY POINTS: It is important to make sure that the hips are not thrust forward, as this can arch the spine and put pressure in the lower back. The movement of tucking the pelvis under is hardly perceptible, but it can be very strong. Do not release the stretch until the full ten breaths in and out are completed. Be sure to maintain the B-Line! This will assist in a stronger stretch. Keep the foot of the supporting left leg at a right angle to the knee so no undue pressure is placed on the toes. Use the tripod position for this foot. You can increase your stretch by using mild pressure of the hands to enhance the tuck, as the muscles may be too tight to achieve this on their own. To achieve an even greater stretch, imagine that the hip-bone of the leg being stretched is drawing strongly up to the rib cage on that side.

CARE: Same as for Thigh Stretch 2. In addition, after stretching each leg, place the hands on the floor to change legs. The closer the knee is to the wall, the better the stretch. If you feel any pain in the knee joint, stop the exercise and try Exercise 11. Keep the hand on the buttock only, not on the lower back.

REPETITIONS: Two sets of ten breaths in and ten breaths out, alternating legs.

BREATHING: Hold the position on the breath in, tuck the pelvis on the breath out.

ADVANCED VERSIONS:
If you feel only a minimal stretch with the above exercise, try the following:

1. Place the supporting leg farther forward and lean the entire body forward away from the wall and heel. Without arching the back, tuck the pelvis in this position. You will feel the stretch higher up the thigh, toward the hipbone.

2. If this is too easy, stay in the forward-leaning position, reach back, and grasp the foot away from the wall toward the buttock. Try to maintain the tuck without arching the back. This should induce an extremely strong stretch toward the top of the thigh.

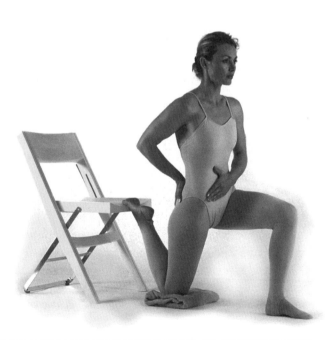

CHAPTER 6

The Routine for Lower Back Pain and Weak Abdominals

Ideally, our muscles

should obey our will.

Reasonably, our will

should not be dominated

by the reflex actions of

our muscles.

J. PILATES

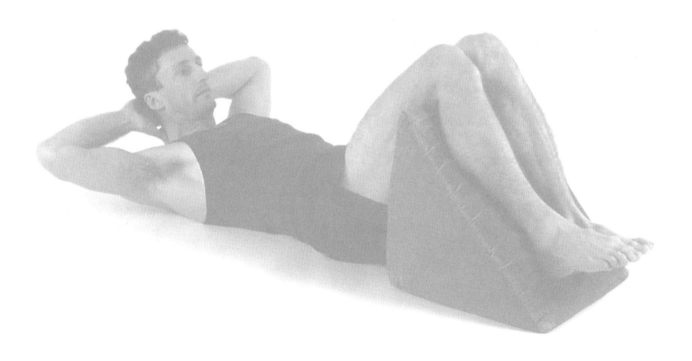

Exercise 14
ONE-LEG LIFTS: SUPINE

ADVANCED: Attempt the same abdominal connection while either extending one leg on the ground or drawing both knees to the chest at the same time without allowing the back to arch.

NOTES

PREREQUISITES: Warm-up stretches.

PURPOSE: To achieve basic abdominal strength for the lower abdominals.

EXERCISE DESCRIPTION:

Starting Position: Lie on your back (supine) with the knees bent at 45 degrees. Without tucking, do the B-Line and place your fingers on the insides of the hipbones. Press firmly.

a) Breathing out, draw the right knee toward your chest without the right buttock lifting off the ground. Do not place any pressure on the floor with the left foot. As the foot is lifted off the floor, you may feel the abdominals push up against the fingers. Draw the abdominals in as hard as you can away from the fingers.

b) Hold the leg toward you for the breath in, then breathe out as you slowly lower the leg to the floor.

KEY POINTS: Sigh on the breath out and flatten the rib cage to the floor.

CARE: If the lower back continues to arch when the leg lifts, place the stationary leg up on a chair.

REPETITIONS: Ten on each leg, alternating after each repetition.

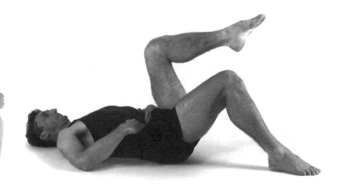

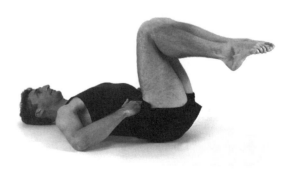

Exercise 15
SLIDING LEG

PREREQUISITES: Warm-up stretches.

PURPOSE: To maintain abdominal connection when the body is lengthening.

EXERCISE DESCRIPTION:

Starting Position: Lie on your back with legs extended and fingers placed on the lower abdominals. Press firmly. Draw these muscles in from the fingers. Put your body in the B-Line.

   a) Breathing out, bend one leg up to your chest, slowly sliding the foot along the floor, intensifying the control from the lower abdominal muscles.

   b) Breathe in as the leg slowly extends away, still drawing the abdominals away from your fingers.

KEY POINTS: Imagine that the abdominal muscles are connected to the thigh and that they are drawing in tighter as you draw the leg toward you. As the leg extends away from you, let the abdominals lengthen and flatten.

CARE: Do not tighten the buttocks. On the breaths in and out, draw the ribs to the hips, breathing into the shoulder blades. Keep the neck lengthened and the shoulders relaxed. If the neck is arched, place a small cushion under the head.

REPETITIONS: Ten on each leg, alternating after each repetition.

VARIATIONS:

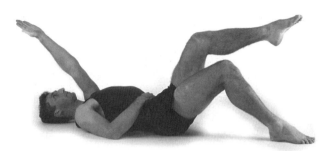

1. *More Challenging:* Start with the right arm on the floor above the head. Breathe in as the right leg draws toward you, while raising the right arm to the ceiling. Extend both the arm and the leg to the floor while maintaining the B-Line and flattening the rib cage to the hips.

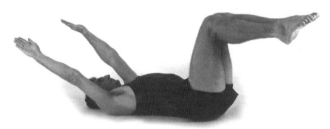

2. *Even More Challenging:* Repeat the preceding variation while using both arms and both legs together, trying to control any arch in the back by maintaining the B-Line and flattening the rib cage on the breath out (extension of the body).

NOTES

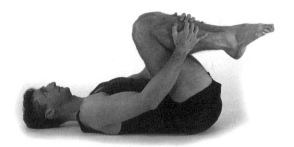

REST POSITION WITH KNEES TO CHEST FOR EXERCISES DONE WHILE LYING ON THE BACK

Lie on your back on a comfortable mat. Draw the knees to the chest and place the hands on the ankles, drawing the heels into the tailbone without lifting the buttocks. Lengthen the neck and press the shoulder blades to the hips. This is the standard position for the start of most exercises that then progress to a contraction position (head forward, shoulder blades off the ground, arms forward past the hips).

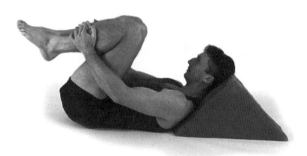

POSITION WITH CUSHIONS FOR ALL EXERCISES

Lie on a large cushion or several pillows with the shoulder blades at the junction of the floor and the cushion. There should be no gap between the back and the floor at any time during the exercise, especially if the arms are raised into the air or behind the head. The head, neck, and chin should be comfortable, with at least a golf-ball space between the chin and the chest at all times. If the knees are raised vertically, the eyes should be focused at a point slightly above the knees.

Exercise 16
PREPARATION WITH CUSHIONS

PREREQUISITES: Warm-up stretches.

PURPOSE: To strengthen and gain control of the abdominals and to feel the entire abdominal section working.

EXERCISE DESCRIPTION:

Starting Position: Lying on the cushion, draw the knees to the chest and hold on to them lightly with your hands.

a) Breathe out as you extend the hands forward past the hips and just off the floor, while extending the legs vertically into the air.

b) Put your body in the B-Line and draw the ribs to the hips.

c) Breathe in as you return to the starting position.

KEY POINTS: Keep the eyes focused above the knees. Be sure to let out a deep sigh. The B-Line should be done hard to connect the abdominals while scooping them for greater effect and support for the lower back.

CARE: Raise the legs only as high as you can without the back arching at all. As you complete more repetitions, the abdominals may weaken and the back take over. Stop at this point.

REPETITIONS: Do ten repetitions. When you first do the exercise, rest for half a second between each repetition to gain continual tone in the muscle. As you become more proficient at this exercise, do not rest at all.

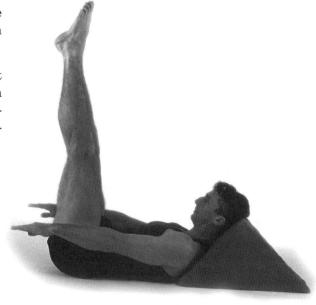

CHAPTER 7

The Basic Routine

Remember, too,

that "Rome was not

built in a day," and that

patience and persistence

are vital qualities in

the ultimate successful

accomplishment of any

worthwhile endeavor.

J. PILATES

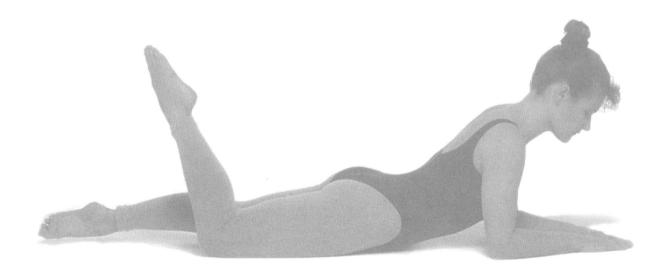

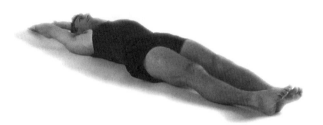

Exercise 17
PREPARATION FOR THE HUNDREDS

PREREQUISITES: Warm-up stretches.

PURPOSE: Abdominal work to control and reduce overarching in the lower back.

EXERCISE DESCRIPTION:

Starting Position: Lie supine on the floor with the arms above the head and the legs together, toes pointed (Figure i).

Figure i

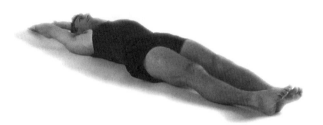

a) Breathe in as you raise the arms to the ceiling and bend the knees, sliding the toes on the ground (Figure ii).

b) Do the B-Line and breathe out as you contract forward, extending the arms past the hips just off the floor and raise the legs vertically (Figure iii). Breathe in as you raise the arms vertically and bend the knees so the toes touch the floor.

c) Breathe out as you extend the arms and legs to the floor to the starting position.

KEY POINTS: Stretch through the fingertips. Slide the toes along the floor, keeping the heels off the floor. Keep the shoulders pressed to the hips at all times.

CARE: Do not jerk up; keep the rhythm smooth during the movement. If the neck starts to strain after several movements, put cushions under the head and take the arms back only as far as is comfortable.

REPETITIONS: Do ten repetitions.

Figure ii

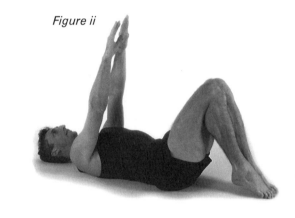

Figure iii

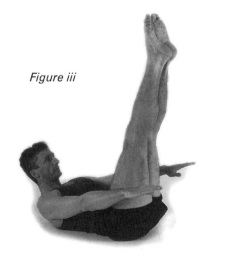

Exercise 18
THE HUNDREDS: BASIC

PREREQUISITES: The Start Stretches (Exercises 3 to 6a).

PURPOSE: To strengthen the abdominal muscles.

EXERCISE DESCRIPTION:

Starting Position: Lie on your back with knees to your chest, hands relaxed on the ankles.

a) Do the B-Line and breathe out as you contract forward. Extended the hands forward through the fingertips, palms down, 6 inches off the floor.

b) Raise your legs vertically into the air, flexing your feet and externally rotating your legs from the thighs. Touch the back of the knees together to stretch the hamstrings and connect the adductors (this will take the pressure off the front of the thighs). Pinch the buttocks slightly.

c) Keeping the eyes on the knees and maintaining the B-Line, breathe in for five seconds and breathe out for five seconds. Repeat ten breaths in and out without resting. (The ten seconds in and out by ten repetitions equals one hundred—hence, the name The Hundreds.)

KEY POINTS: Keep the rib cage drawn to the hips at all times, shoulder blades off the mat and relaxed forward, eyes on the knees. If the shoulders drop back on the breath in, contract forward farther on the breath in. Scoop the abdominals. If you do not feel the abdominals while doing this exercise, then attempt the intermediate Hundreds.

CARE: If the back arches or strains, turn the legs in and bend the knees slightly. When the knees are bent, keep the heels in a vertical line with the buttocks to keep the back flat. If you feel the neck strain, place a cushion under the head, raise the head on each breath out, and rest on the breath in, remembering to keep the B-Line even in the rest position. As the neck becomes stronger, raise the head up for two breaths, and so on.

To assist in maintaining the B-Line, place a small weight on the lower abdominals and draw the abdominals away from the weight, especially on the breath in. When the weight no longer moves, remove it.

REPETITIONS: Two sets of ten breaths in and ten breaths out. Take no more than a ten-second rest between each set.

NOTES

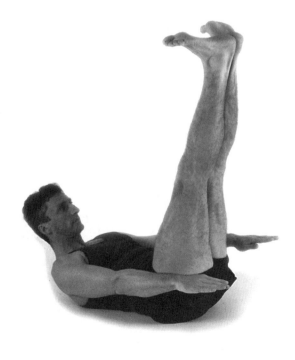

Exercise 19-1
THE HUNDREDS: INTERMEDIATE

NOTES

PREREQUISITES: Warm-up stretches and the ability to do two sets of basic Hundreds comfortably.

PURPOSE: To strengthen the abdominals by moving the body's center of gravity.

EXERCISE DESCRIPTION: Start in the same position as for the basic Hundreds. Lower the legs until you feel the back is just about to lift off the mat, making sure the abdominals do not lift even one millimeter (think of a greyhound's stomach). Do the B-Line. Breathe in ten times and out ten times.

KEY POINTS: The back must remain flat throughout the exercise. Keep the shoulder blades just off the floor at all times.

CARE: If the abdominals rise higher than the level of the hips and ribs, raise the legs higher and scoop the stomach. Try to increase the B-Line before every breath in.

REPETITIONS: Two sets of ten breaths.

ADVANCED: To connect the lower abdominals more specifically, even while using the B-Line, keep the legs at a low angle (lower than 45 degrees), and without moving the angle of the legs, try to lift your buttocks off the floor. They will not actually lift a noticeable distance, but you should feel the immediate, strong connection of the lower abdominals. Keep your buttocks lifted for the whole set.

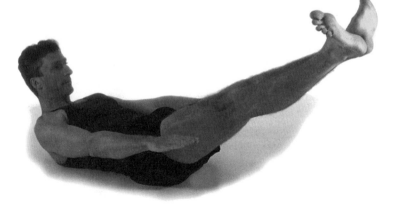

Exercise 19-2
PERCUSSION BREATHING

This exercise follows the same routine as the preceding one, with the following addition: Keep the legs parallel, with the toes softly pointed. Pump the hands up and down a few inches, each pump taking half a second. Breathe in for five pumps and breathe out for five pumps until you have completed one hundred pumps (or ten breaths in and ten breaths out).

Instead of a smooth five seconds of breathing in, the breathing should be done as five individual breaths in (or out) until full capacity (or deflation) is achieved. This gives a percussion effect to the breathing, and it can increase the effect on the abdominals even more. Squeeze a thin pad between the knees for more abdominal effect.

CARE: If you find that this exercise is working in the neck and not very strongly in the abdominals, revert to the basic Hundreds until the abdominals are stronger.

Exercise 20
SINGLE LEG STRETCH

PREREQUISITES: The Start Stretches (Exercises 3 to 6a).

PURPOSE: To mobilize the hip and knee joints, control the abdominals, and increase coordination.

EXERCISE DESCRIPTION:

Starting Position: Lie flat on your back, with both knees to the chest.

 a) Breathe out as you contract forward, placing the right hand on the right ankle and the left hand on the right knee, elbows raised.

 b) Extend the left leg away from the body in line with the hip and as low to the floor as possible, without the back arching. As the leg extends, turn it out and stretch through the point of the foot.

 c) Do the B-Line and scoop the stomach. Breathe in as you change legs, keeping the outside hand on the ankle (left hand, left ankle), and draw the left knee to the left shoulder.

KEY POINTS: Keep the shoulders relaxed, chin slightly off the chest. Do the B-Line before changing legs, and keep the ribs as close to the hips as possible. Use the hands as a guide; do not use them to pull on the leg. When extending the leg, try to feel as if the inner thigh were squeezing a cushion. When extending the leg from the bent position, stretch through the toe along the line of the final position of the leg (do not extend into the air and then lower the leg to the ground). Keep the shoulders square at all times by pressing both elbows toward the hips.

CARE: If the neck starts to strain, place a cushion under the head and shoulders.

REPETITIONS: One set of ten repetitions, alternating legs.

VARIATIONS:

 1. Instead of holding on with the hands, place the wrists over the knee and ankle, with the fingers extended to the far walls. This action will ease the knee closer to the shoulder and reduce any excessive neck and shoulder work.

 2. After six repetitions, extend the arms past the hips and continue to alternate the legs. Try to draw the knees back as close to the shoulders as before, on their own. Repeat for ten repetitions. Feel the abdominals.

NOTES

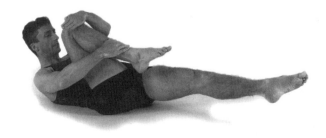

Exercise 21
DOUBLE LEG STRETCH: BASIC

This exercise may appear confusing because of the amount of instruction. Please persevere: it will be worth it!

PREREQUISITES: Preparation for the Hundreds (Exercise 17), The Hundreds: Basic (Exercise 18).

PURPOSE: To strengthen the abdominals while moving the body's center of gravity. To mobilize the shoulder joints. To coordinate breathing and arm and leg movement with abdominal control.

EXERCISE DESCRIPTION:

Starting Position: Lie on your back on the floor, knees comfortably bent to the chest, slightly apart, toes pointed and touching, and hands on the ankles (or shins, whichever does not hunch the shoulders). Draw the ankles to the buttocks. Place your head on a cushion if required (Figure i).

a) Do the B-Line and breathe out as you contract forward. Extend the arms forward through the fingertips, 6 inches off the floor. On the same breath out, extend the legs into the air (flexed and turned out), as low to the floor as is comfortable. Keep the back flat and scoop the stomach. Press through the heels, and squeeze the inner thighs (Figure ii).

b) Breathe in as you reach through the fingers and extend the arms to a vertical position to the ceiling (don't hunch the shoulders). Hold the position for one second and do the B-Line harder (Figure iii).

c) Keeping the B-Line, breathe out as you extend the arms behind the head (scraping the ears) in a big circle around and back to their starting position by the hips. Draw the ribs to the hips even tighter (Figure iv).

d) Breathe in as you return to your starting position. Rest for only half a second before repeating the movement.

KEY POINTS: As the arms move from the vertical position to behind the head, ensure that the ribs stay toward the hips. This movement should always be done on a breath out, depressing the rib cage. Press through the heels as far as you can. Externally rotate the legs as much as possible. Stretch through the tips of the fingers at all times, making sure not to hunch the shoulders. Do not allow the shoulder blades to lower to the floor on the arm circle.

CARE: If the neck feels any pressure, keep the head on a high cushion at all times. If the back begins to arch after several movements, raise the legs to a higher position so that the small of the back stays flat on the floor. Take a deep, long sigh out as the arms move (float) behind the head.

REPETITIONS: One set of ten.

BREATHING: As you contract forward, raising the legs into the air, breathe in as you raise the arms from 6 inches off the floor to the vertical position. Breathe out as you take the arms behind the head and complete the circle to the hips, and breathe in as you return to the rest position.

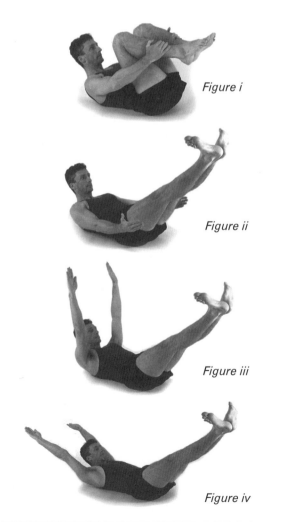

Figure i

Figure ii

Figure iii

Figure iv

Exercise 22
SINGLE LEG CIRCLES 1

PREREQUISITES: The Start Stretches (Exercises 3 to 6a).

PURPOSE: To isolate the adductor muscle and mobilize the hip joint.

EXERCISE DESCRIPTION:

Starting Position: Lie on the floor with both knees bent, thighs at 45 degrees. Place the hands on the floor, palms down, elbows slightly bent, and thumb and index fingers just touching the buttock on each side. Do the B-Line. Raise the right leg to the ceiling, with the foot pointed, and turn out the leg. Press the right buttock into the mat, and press the fingers of the right hand against the right adductor muscle close to the groin to connect the muscle.

a) Making a counterclockwise circle, breathe out as you lower the leg, allowing the abdominals to lengthen. Extend through the toes as if you were drawing a circle on the ceiling with them. Keep the hip pressed into the mat (the circle is actually a D shape with a straight line up the middle to start).

b) Breathe in as you raise the leg to the vertical position, maintaining the B-Line.

KEY POINTS: Do not allow the buttock of the resting leg to lift off the fingers at all; keep them just touching. Feel the inner thigh (adductor) muscle making the circle by pressing against the fingers to establish the connection (eventually, remove the fingers). Keep the circle high and small to start.

CARE: Do not push the supporting leg into the ground. This will place pressure into the lower back and raise the buttock, and it can place the pelvis out of alignment.

REPETITIONS: Do six circles in one direction, then change legs. Repeat the circles in the other direction.

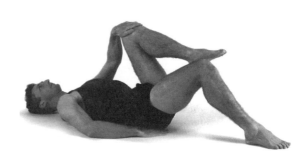

**EASIER VARIATION:
HAND ON THE KNEE**

If this exercise is too difficult to perform for more than four repetitions, then try the following: Instead of extending a straight leg to the ceiling, bend the knee and place the hand on the knee. Make a circle only as far as the hand will allow, away from the body. Imagine you are stirring a pot with the thigh bone. Gradually extend the leg into the air, keeping the hand on the knee until the leg is almost fully extended.

NOTES

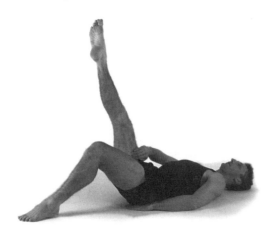

Exercise 23
SIDE TO SIDE

PREREQUISITES: Warm-up stretches, and no major back problems.

PURPOSE: To strengthen the obliques while in an elongated position. To provide abdominal support for the back while in rotation.

EXERCISE DESCRIPTION:

Starting Position: Lie on your back with the knees drawn to the chest so they are above the lower ribs. Squeeze a thin pad between the knees. Keep the calves parallel to the floor and the feet pointed. Place the arms by your sides with the palms up.

a) Over to the side: Do the B-Line and breathe out as you take both knees over to the right side, but only halfway to the floor. Keep the opposite shoulder blade on the floor at all times. Start by peeling the right hip off the floor, keeping the knees level with each other and in line with the ribs.

b) Return to center: Do not press your right arm on the floor to assist the body to return to the center. First do the B-Line more and then breathe in as you slowly roll the left rib cage to the floor, imprinting the spine onto the floor from the shoulder blade to the hip. As you begin to roll the spine to the floor, keep the knees in line with the ribs.

c) Without stopping, breathe out as you flow the movement to the left side.

KEY POINTS: Press the knees together. Keep the feet parallel to the floor at all times. Keep the shoulders relaxed on the floor. Try not to move them. When comfortable (stable) with the movement, turn the head in the opposite direction to the knees to rotate throughout the length of the spine. This exercise should be felt in the abdominals only, never in the back.

CARE: When taking the knees over to the side, make sure they do not twist at the hips. Both knees must move together so that the lower back does not twist. When you return to the center, if the hip is pulled over first, the back will tend to do the work, defeating the purpose of the exercise.

REPETITIONS: One set of ten repetitions on each side.

NOTES

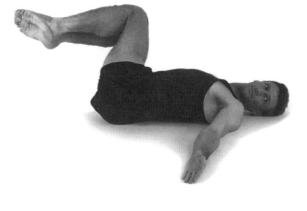

Exercise 24
STOMACH STRETCH

NOTES

PREREQUISITE: The Hundreds: Basic (Exercise 18).

PURPOSE: To strengthen the abdominals in elongation, and to strengthen the back.

EXERCISE DESCRIPTION:

Starting Position: Lie on your stomach (prone) on the floor with your arms stretched above the head, legs extended hip-distance apart, toes pointed. Rest your forehead on the ground or on a cushion to keep the neck in line with the upper back.

a) Do the B-Line and slightly tighten your buttocks. Breathe out as you extend the left arm 2 inches off the ground. Imagine someone is holding your wrist and lengthening the limb out of the socket, without hunching the level line of the shoulders.

b) Breathe in as you keep the lengthened feeling and return to lightly touch the floor, scooping the abdominals even more.

c) Breathe out as you extend the other arm.

KEY POINTS: Keep the B-Line so that a ruler could easily slide between the mat and your stomach at all times. Elongate the back of the neck, and keep the shoulder blades pressed to the hips.

CARE: If the abdominals feel as if they were resting on the floor, the back muscles will start to do the work. Keep them supported by the abdominal contraction. If the back does begin to take over, stop. Attempt one more stretch each day with an increase in abdominal work.

REPETITIONS: One set of ten alternating lifts.

BASIC/INTERMEDIATE VARIATION: Alternate Leg Lifts.

Follow the same procedure as in the preceding exercise, but this time use the legs instead of the arms.

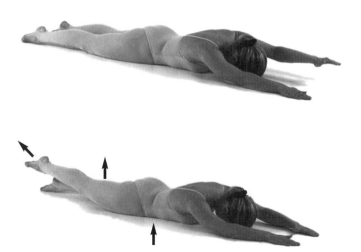

Exercise 25
THE PERFECT ABDOMINAL CURL

PREREQUISITES: The Start Stretches (Exercises 3 to 6a).

PURPOSE: To provide basic abdominal strength for all exercises.

EXERCISE DESCRIPTION:

Starting Position: Lie on your back on the floor, with the knees together, bent at 45 degrees, so the feet are approximately 10–12 inches from the buttocks. The entire back must be flat. Place your hands where they are most comfortable, either behind the head so they are on the opposite shoulders to support the neck, or with fingers interlocked behind the head with elbows wide open (photo), or with the arms crossed on the chest.

a) Do the B-Line and, breathing out, draw the ribs as close as possible to the hips in the same horizontal plane as the floor until the shoulder blades come off the ground. Scoop the abdominals (imagine a greyhound's stomach).

b) Breathe in and slowly release the abdominals 10 percent or allow the torso to lower so that the shoulder blades almost touch the floor.

Without stopping, repeat ten times.

KEY POINTS: If the hands are behind the head, keep the elbows wide open. The arms are there to support the head, not to pull it forward. Keep the chin off the chest and the eyes focused just above the knees. Imagine using the area between the ribs and the hips as a bellows that you close on the breath out and release on the breath in.

CARE: Contract forward (draw the ribs to the hips) without the ribs lifting above the level of the hips, as this can bunch the abdominals out. Concentrating on drawing the ribs to the hips should ease some strain on the neck. It is this movement that connects the abdominals, not the lift of the head, neck, and shoulders. If the neck strains, stop. Move smoothly, without momentum or any jerky movements. If the back is arched, place the feet on a chair with the knees above the navel.

REPETITIONS: Up to three sets of ten to twelve repetitions.

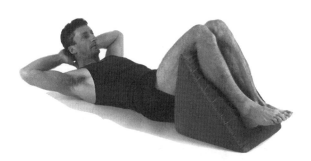

VARIATIONS FOR GREATER ABDOMINAL CONNECTION:

1. Flex the feet so that you are lightly balancing on the heels.

2. Place the legs over high cushions so when they are relaxed, the thighs do not flop open and the heels do not touch the ground. This position greatly reduces the connection of the front of the thighs (quadriceps) and the inner thighs (adductors). Keep the thighs relaxed during the entire set. This works the abdominals more specifically with less strain on the lower back.

NOTES

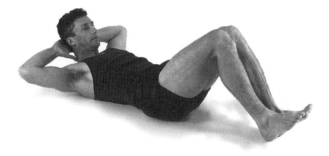

Exercise 26-1
ANKLE WEIGHTS: OUTER THIGH (ABDUCTOR)

PREREQUISITE: None.

PURPOSE: To strengthen and tone the hip by working the outer part and the back of the thighs.

EXERCISE DESCRIPTION:
This exercise may be done with any of the following:

- No ankle weights (the weight of the leg may be sufficient to begin)

- A 2 lb. weight on each leg

- A 4 or 5 lb. weight on each leg (advanced and men only)

Starting Position: Lie on the right side with the body in a straight line. As in all routines done lying on the side, you should lie with your back against a wall to ensure correct spinal posture. Do not lean against the wall—just use it as a guide to maintain a straight back. Place the right arm under the head, extended in a line with the body, with the palm facing upward. Bend the right leg up to 45 degrees with the foot remaining in line with the body. Bring the straight, left leg 6 inches forward to keep the back flat. Flex the left foot and raise the leg off the ground 6 inches.

The following are important for the perfect execution of the exercise:

a) Press the left hip away from the left rib with the left hand so that the left hip sits on top of the right hip. The hips are now aligned vertically. Do the B-Line. Imagine that the weight is on the outside of the thigh about 6 inches from the hip joint.

b) Breathe out and, lengthening through the heel, raise the leg approximately 6–12 inches maximum above the height of the hip. You should feel the outer thigh of the leg working strongly.

c) Breathing in, lower the leg to just below hip level before repeating. Do not rest the leg on the floor.

KEY POINTS: Keep the hips aligned. If the top hip continually moves into the waist with the movement of the leg, the exercise becomes less effective.

CARE: Be sure to maintain the B-Line. If the back tends to arch, tuck the pelvis so that the back is touching, but not pressing against, the wall. As the repetitions increase, focus on lengthening through the heel. Do not hunch the top shoulder or rotate it forward while pressing the top hip away from the rib cage. (An alternative to pressing the top hip away is to place the left hand, palm up, between the right side of the waist and the floor, closer to the hip. Now create a gap between the palm of the hand and the waist, without hunching the shoulder. As the leg lifts, attempt to increase the size of this gap. If the waist touches the hand every time the leg is raised, the leg is being raised too high, causing the hip to move.)

REPETITIONS: Ten to twenty on each leg.

ADVANCED: Bend the knee so that it is "unlocked" for all the repetitions.

NOTES

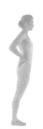

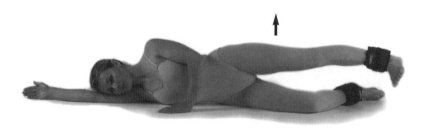

Exercise 26-2
ANKLE WEIGHTS: INNER THIGH (ADDUCTOR)

PREREQUISITE: None.

PURPOSE: To strengthen, while lengthening, the inner thigh.

EXERCISE DESCRIPTION:

Starting Position: Lie on you right side and place a high cushion by the hip against the abdomen. Bend the left leg and rest it on top of the cushion, with the right arm extended under the head and the left hand relaxed on the floor. Draw the right leg forward so the foot is 12 inches away from the wall behind you. Keep the right leg parallel and straight with the foot pointed. If you don't have a cushion, place the leg as in the photo.

    a) Imagine the weight is sitting high on the inner right thigh between the knee and the groin. Do the B-Line, and as you breathe out, raise the right inner thigh as high as possible without moving any other part of the body.

    b) Still lengthening through the toe, breathe in as the leg is lowered and lightly touches the floor before repeating the lift. Do not rest between repetitions.

KEY POINTS: Do not place any pressure on the cushion to lift the lower leg. Do the B-Line on the lifting and lowering of the leg.

CARE: Keep the bottom leg forward of the body. If the leg straightens in line with the body, the back will tend to arch and lessen the work of the abdominals and the inner thigh. If the bottom hip is uncomfortable, lie on a flat cushion.

REPETITIONS: One set of ten to twenty repetitions.

ADVANCED:

Do one or both of the following:

1. Unlock the knee and continue to lengthen through the foot.

2. Turn out the lower leg from the inner thigh, without moving the hips from their vertical position.

NOTES

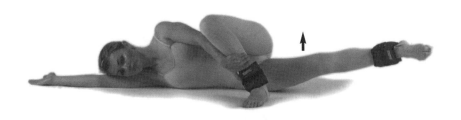

Exercise 26-3
ANKLE WEIGHTS: OUTER THIGH FLEXION (ABDUCTOR)

PREREQUISITE: Ankle Weights: Outer Thigh (Exercise 26-1).

PURPOSE: To strengthen the outer thigh when the leg is at a right angle to the body.

EXERCISE DESCRIPTION:
This exercise may be done with any of the following:

- No ankle weights (the weight of the leg may be sufficient to begin)

- A 2 lb. weight on each leg

- A 4 or 5 lb. weight on each leg (advanced and men only)

Starting Position: For this exercise, lie on your right side with your back against a wall to ensure correct spinal posture. Do not lean against the wall—just use it as a guide to maintain a straight back. Place the right arm under the head, extended in a line with the body, with the palm facing upward. Bend the right leg up to 45 degrees with the foot remaining in line with the body. Flex the left foot and raise the leg off the ground 6 inches.

a) Do the B-Line and take the left leg as far forward as possible, at hip level, so that the top knee is above the bent knee. (If the top leg can go farther forward and you feel unbalanced, bend the bottom leg higher so the knees remain vertically aligned with each other.) Breathe out and lift the outer thigh so that the foot rises up to 6 inches higher than the level of the hip. Do not lift from the foot.

b) Breathe in as the left leg lowers just below hip height. Repeat.

KEY POINTS: Attempt to keep the top hip aligned with the bottom one. The angle of the leg to the body will generally determine the movement in the hip joint. The farther away the leg is from the right angle, the more stable the hip will be. Press the left hip away from the left rib with the left hand so that it sits on top of the right hip. The hips are now aligned vertically.

CARE: This is a difficult exercise. You may not be able to complete the same number of repetitions of this as you did of the previous two ankle-weight exercises. Do not overdo it.

REPETITIONS: Ten to twenty on each side.

ADVANCED

1. Unlock the top knee.

2. Turn the leg in to the floor from the thigh without moving the hip.

NOTES

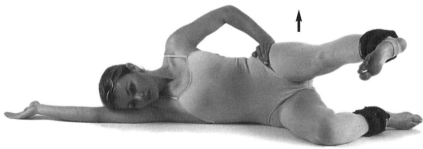

Exercise 27
BACK OF THE THIGH: HAMSTRING/BUTTOCKS

PREREQUISITES: Ankle Weights (Exercises 26-1 to 26-3).

PURPOSE: To strengthen the hamstring and tone and tighten the buttocks.

EXERCISE DESCRIPTION:

Starting Position: Lie prone (on the stomach) with a flat cushion under the abdominals (between the ribs and the hips), with the forehead rested on the hands and the legs extended, turned out with the feet flexed. Place a thick pad in between the legs and tightly into the crotch.

a) Do the B-Line and breathe out as you raise the legs 2 inches and squeeze the pad. Try to touch your knees together. Keep the abdominals drawn up away from the cushion. Do not allow the hips to lift off the floor.

b) Breathe in and release 10 percent before repeating.

KEY POINTS: Keep the B-Line to support the lower back. Do not hunch the shoulders or put pressure on the elbows.

CARE: To avoid arching the back, do not raise the legs higher than 2 inches. If the knees do touch, place a thicker pad in the groin.

REPETITIONS: Two sets of ten to twenty repetitions.

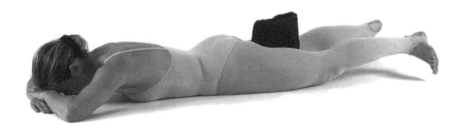

PREREQUISITE: None.

PURPOSE: To strengthen and mobilize the arms, chest, back, and neck.

EXERCISE DESCRIPTION: Base the weights you use on your strength. You can use heavier weights for Exercise 28-1, as no rotation of the joint is involved. If you do this exercise at home, you can use cans of beans in place of weights. All of these arm weight exercises are done lying on the back (supine).

KEY POINTS: Lie on the floor or on a narrow bench, knees bent at a 45-degree angle. Maintain the B-Line. Do not allow the back to arch at any time. However, do not excessively tilt the pelvis or put pressure on the feet to force the back down.

CARE: Raise the arms vertically to the ceiling above the chest (not above the face), fingers extended (to obtain maximum elongation from the shoulder joint). The hands should be placed shoulder distance apart, palms facing each other.

Do not round the shoulders off the floor or hunch the shoulders to the ears.

"Unlock" the elbows, but continue to elongate through the length of the arm and out of the extended fingers.

Keep the neck long and the shoulder blades always pressed toward the hips. If the neck is arched, or if there is a large gap between the back of the neck and the bench, place a cushion under the head for more comfort.

For all the arm weight exercises, it is essential to imagine that the weight is near the top of the arm, about 6 inches from the shoulder. This makes it easier to lift the weight and to connect the upper arm muscles.

Breathe into the chest and, on the breath out, flatten the ribs to the hips. By pressing the ribs to the hips, this has the dual benefit of connecting the upper abdominals as well as stabilizing the middle and upper back. (Imagine that a slab of concrete is pressing on your chest on the breath out.)

If lying on a bench, do not allow the arms to drop below the level of the bench. If lying on the floor, do not let the weights or arms rest on the floor at any time.

If you have any "clicking" or strain in the shoulder joints, reduce the range of the movement.

Maintain the B-Line at all times.

NOTES

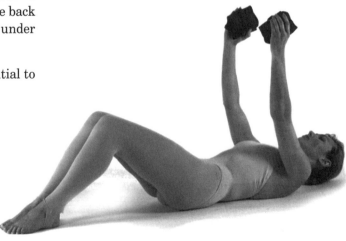

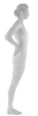

Exercise 28-1
OPENING ARMS

PREREQUISITE & PURPOSE: Same as for Exercise 28.

EXERCISE DESCRIPTION:

a) Imagine that a huge beach ball is being pumped up between your arms and, breathing in, resist as the arms are being pressed open to the sides.

b) Breathing out on the upward movement, squeeze the air out of the beach ball. Feel the chest muscles (pectoral muscles) doing the work to raise the arms to the ceiling (imagine that you have a pencil on your breastbone and are trying to squeeze it with your chest muscles). Alternatively, get a friend to gently press against the pectoral muscles as you press against their fingers when closing.

KEY POINTS & CARE: Same as for Exercise 28.

REPETITIONS: One set of up to twenty repetitions.

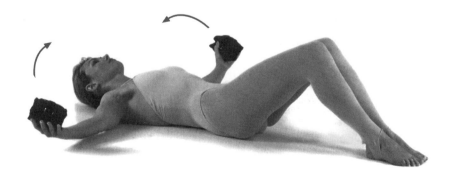

Exercise 28-2
ALTERNATING ARMS

PREREQUISITE & PURPOSE: Same as for Exercise 28.

EXERCISE DESCRIPTION:

a) Breathing out, extend the right arm down to your right foot and at the same time extend the left arm to your left ear and to a point above your head, flattening the rib cage.

Do not hunch the left shoulder. Keep a gap between the left arm and the left ear. Do not rest the weight above the head. If the left arm does not extend toward the level of the ear without the rib cage lifting, slowly release the left chest muscle.

b) Before returning to the upright position, do the B-Line more, flatten the rib cage, and, breathing in, lengthen the arms to the ceiling. Lengthen the left arm by engaging the muscles in the back of the upper arm (the triceps). To connect this muscle and avoid shoulder strain, imagine squashing an orange under the armpit, or get a friend to gently apply pressure halfway between the elbow and the shoulder and press against this.

If the left shoulder is raised slightly toward the ear, press it toward the hip before raising the arm to the ceiling. You should then get a better connection both above and below the shoulder joint (the latissimus dorsi will connect).

Lengthen both arms to the starting position and, without stopping in the vertical position, alternate the movement.

KEY POINTS & CARE: Same as for Exercise 28.

REPETITIONS: One set of ten on each side, alternating sides.

NOTES

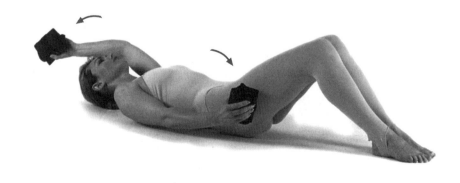

PREREQUISITE & PURPOSE: Same as for Exercise 28.

EXERCISE DESCRIPTION:

Starting Position: Lightly touch the fingertips (or knuckles) of each hand together above the chest with the elbows slightly bend outward.

a) Do the B-Line and, breathing out, extend both arms above the head to a point where the ribs do not lift, the back does not arch, and the shoulders do not hunch.

b) Do not rest the arms. Flatten the ribs to the hips, and press the shoulder blades to the hips.

c) Breathe in as the arms float back up to the ceiling. Imagine squashing oranges under the armpits to connect the upper back of the arms and the latissimum dorsi.

Repeat without stopping.

KEY POINTS & CARE: Same as for Exercise 28.

REPETITIONS: One set of ten.

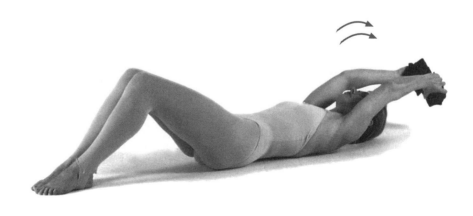

Exercise 28-4
ARM CIRCLES

PREREQUISITE & PURPOSE: Same as for Exercise 28.

EXERCISE DESCRIPTION:

a) Do the B-Line and, breathing in, extend both hands down toward the heels, palms facing each other. Do not allow the arms to go below bench level.

b) Turn the palms up to the ceiling, and, breathing out, extend the arms out to the sides just above bench or floor level until they reach as close to the ears as is comfortable.

c) At this point, keep moving, palms facing inward, and breathe in as the arms extend to the ceiling and continue down to the feet. If the shoulder joints are tight, you may make the circle smaller.

Remember to squeeze the imaginary oranges under the armpits when raising the arms from above the head to the ceiling and to the feet. Try not to bend the elbows any farther than the "unlocked" position for the entire routine.

KEY POINTS & CARE: Same as for Exercise 28.

REPETITIONS: One set of ten in one direction, then one set of ten in the other direction. Always start the circles with the movement to the heels first (inward circle).

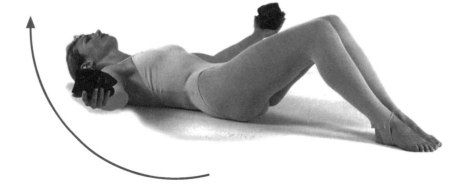

Exercise 29-1
ARM SWINGS: ALTERNATING

PREREQUISITE: None.

PURPOSE: To mobilize the shoulder joints, stretch and open the chest (pectorals), and improve thoracic and cervical posture.

EXERCISE DESCRIPTION:

Starting Position: Stand upright on the tripods of the feet, sideways to a mirror, feet placed hip-distance apart.

a) Do the B-Line and raise the arms up to shoulder level, with the right palm down and the left palm up. Lengthen through the fingertips.

b) Breathe out as you extend the right arm to the ceiling and the left arm to the floor so both palms are facing forward. Do not hunch the right shoulder. Lengthen through the crown of the head. Flatten the ribs to an imaginary wall behind you on the breath out. This will stabilize the thoracic area and help stretch the chest muscles.

c) Continue to take the arms past the (vertical) line of the body. Look in the mirror to ensure that the back is not arching. Imagine you are standing against a wall and the gap between the wall and the lower back cannot increase. Hold the B-Line as firmly as possible.

d) Breathe in as the arms lengthen forward to the shoulder-level position, rotate the arms and hands so the right palm is up and the left palm is down, and continue moving the arms, right arm to the floor and left arm to the ceiling.

KEY POINTS: Maintain the tripod position and the B-Line. Keep the ribs as flat as possible to the hips to prevent them from protruding forward and arching the back. Lengthen through the fingertips.

CARE: Keep the neck long and upright, so it does not crane forward as the arms stretch past the vertical line. Do not hunch the shoulders.

REPETITIONS: One set of ten repetitions on each side, alternating sides.

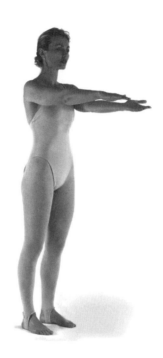

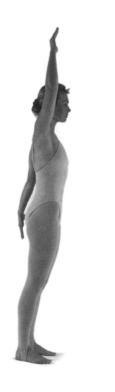

Exercise 29-2
ARM SWINGS: CHEST EXPANSION

PREREQUISITE & PURPOSE: Same as for Exercise 29-1.

EXERCISE DESCRIPTION:

The extended arms start at navel level with the palms up to the ceiling.

a) Breathe out as the arms open up at a 45-degree angle and back behind the head at head level. Feel the stretch across the chest.

b) Breathe in as the arms return to the starting position.

KEY POINTS: Same as for Exercise 29-1.

CARE: As you raise the arms to the ceiling, press the shoulder blades to the floor. Do not jut the chin out.

REPETITIONS: One set of ten repetitions.

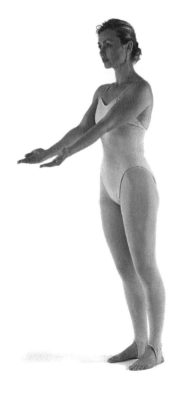 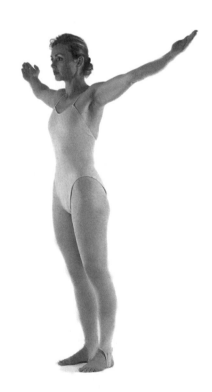

PREREQUISITES: Exercises 28-1 and 28-2.

PURPOSE: To open the chest fully, stretch the pectoral muscles, and improve rotation of the shoulder joints.

EXERCISE DESCRIPTION:

Starting Position: Facing a mirror, do the B-Line and hold on to a pole, broomstick, or Thera-band at shoulder level, hands comfortably wide apart. Hold the pole with only the thumb and forefinger wrapped around it. The other fingers remain extended, in order to prevent torsion in the wrist joint and straining of the neck once the movement has started.

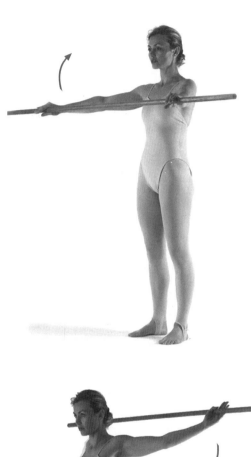

a) Lengthening the pole in front of you as if your shoulders were the radius of a circle, breathe in and raise the pole to the ceiling without hunching the shoulders.

b) Breathe out as the pole lengthens behind the shoulders and down to the floor. Do not bend the elbows. If they, or the shoulders or chest, are too tight, widen your hold on the pole. Lengthen the neck to the ceiling. Do not jut the chin forward.

c) Hold the position with the pole behind your buttocks for the breath in. Do the B-Line and breathe out as you once again press the pole behind the shoulders to the far wall, up to the ceiling and forward to shoulder level.

KEY POINTS: Look in the mirror to ensure that the pole is always parallel to the floor. Maintain the tripod position at all times; do not rock onto the toes or heels at any time.

CARE: Do not crane the neck forward. Do not hold the breath. Press the shoulders to the hips at all times.

REPETITIONS: Ten repetitions (backward and forward is one repetition).

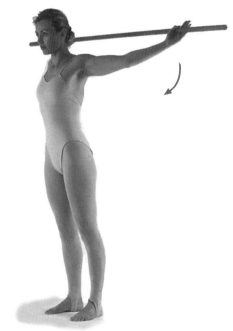

CHAPTER 8

The Intermediate Routine

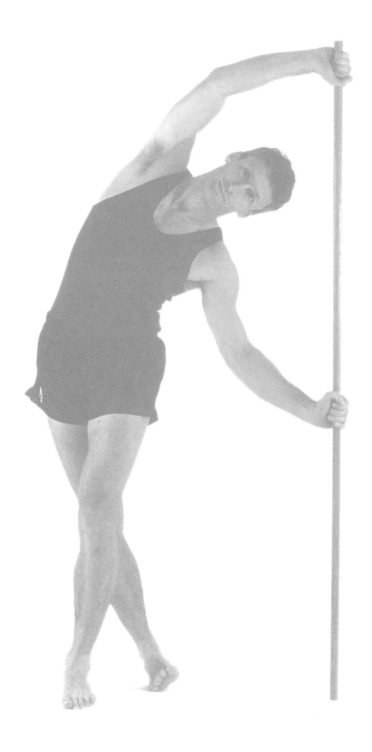

Correctly executed
and mastered to the
point of subconscious
reaction, these exercises
will reflect grace and
balance in your
routine activities.

J. PILATES

Exercise 31
THE HUNDREDS: ALTERNATING LEGS

PREREQUISITE: The Hundreds: Basic (Exercise 18).

PURPOSE: To work each side of the abdominals separately.

EXERCISE DESCRIPTION:

Starting Position: Lie on your back with the legs drawn to the chest, and hold on to the ankles, resting your head on the floor and keeping the neck long. Contract forward (head and shoulders forward, eyes on the knees, ribs drawn to the hips). Extend the legs vertically into the air, feet pointed, legs turned out.

a) Extend the arms through the fingertips several inches off the floor and press the shoulder blades toward the hips. Do the B-Line and breathe out as you flex the foot and lower the right leg down as far to the floor as you can without arching the back. Leave the left leg in the air, drawing it slightly closer to the chest.

b) Do the B-Line more and breathe in as you point the right foot and raise the leg back to the vertical position. Change legs.

KEY POINTS: As the leg lowers, draw the ribs to the hips even closer to counteract any drop of the shoulders. Keep the shoulder blades raised off the floor when raising the leg back to the vertical position. Ensure that the vertical leg is totally straight and turned out, with the foot pointed.

CARE: Do not lower the leg too low if the back lifts the slightest amount. Lengthen the abdominals and allow the thigh muscles to stretch to achieve a controlled lowering of the leg—imagine that the hip joint is opening like a hinge.

REPETITIONS: Five to ten repetitions for each leg.

NOTES

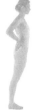

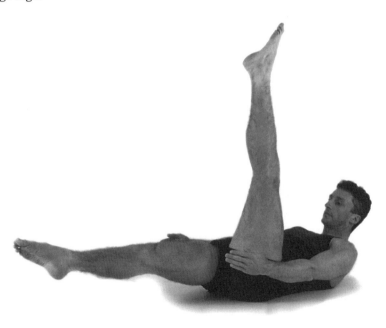

Exercise 32
COORDINATION

PREREQUISITE: The Hundreds: Basic (Exercise 18).

PURPOSE: To coordinate the arms and legs with the breath. To work the adductors, shoulders, upper back, and abdominals.

EXERCISE DESCRIPTION:

Starting Position: Lie on your back, with the knees comfortably to your chest, tailbone on the mat, hands on the knees, and elbows bent.

a) Do the B-Line and breathe out as you contract forward, extending the arms through the fingertips and the legs forward as low as you can without the back arching (legs parallel, with toes softly pointed).

b) Hold the breath as you rapidly open and close the legs once, just wider than shoulder distance, attempting to connect the inner thighs for this movement.

c) Breathe in as you return to the starting position for half a second before repeating.

KEY POINTS: Stretch through the toes as far as you can, even when opening and closing the legs. When returning to the resting position, draw the knees to the chest (rather than dropping the feet to the bottom). Keep the B-Line even when returning to the resting position. Do not allow the abdominals to rest until all repetitions are completed. Squeeze the inner thighs until the final repetition is complete.

CARE: Complete only the number of repetitions required to feel the abdominals working, without feeling any strain in any other part of the body. Focus mentally on every movement of the arms, head, neck, shoulders, legs, and inner thighs, as well as the breathing. Try to feel every fiber of muscle working on the contraction forward as well as on the return to the resting position.

REPETITIONS: One set of ten.

NOTES

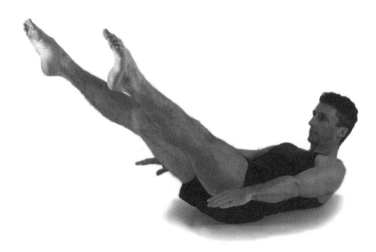

PREREQUISITES: The Start Stretches (Exercises 3 to 6a), the Perfect Abdominal Curl (Exercise 25).

PURPOSE: To strengthen the abdominals and stretch the back.

EXERCISE DESCRIPTION:

Starting Position: Hold on to a short pole (a small towel stretched between your hands will do). Lie on your back on a mat, arms above your head on the floor, elbows extended, legs straight, pressing through your heels.

a) Do the B-Line and take a long breath in as you raise the arms to the ceiling and bring them down to your thighs, flatten the ribs to the floor, and start to roll the chin to the chest.

b) Breathe out and draw the rib cage to the hips. Continue rolling the head and shoulders off the floor in a smooth movement. Continue to roll each vertebra off the mat, at the same time pressing your back into the mat as you peel your spine off the floor.

c) Reach forward as far as you can, lengthening your chest toward your knees and the crown of your head to your toes. Hold this position and take a deep breath into your back.

d) Still reaching the arms toward the feet and pressing through the heels, breathe out as you roll back. Start by sinking into the hips and imprinting the spine back on the mat until the arms are above the head on the floor. Maintain your B-Line at all times.

KEY POINTS: Take 75 percent of your breath out in the first 25 percent of the movement or when the head and shoulders are lifting off the floor. On the return movement, take 75 percent of the breath out in the first 25 percent of the movement after sinking into the hips. If the lungs are too full of air, the back may move as a stiff block, rather than rolling, as it should. It will be easier

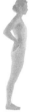

to contract the abdominal area correctly if the lungs are emptying themselves during the roll of the body. Keep reaching forward along the pole on the way up as if someone were pulling the pole forward for you. On the way down, lean forward as if someone were pulling you to your toes as you roll down. This has the effect of opening up your back.

CARE: If the spine is not rolling smoothly all the way (up or down), bend the knees, planting the heels into the ground, and roll through the hips continually on the roll down. Maintain the B-Line. If, on the roll up, the torso lifts rather than rolls, bend the knees more or place light weights on your feet. Engage the hip flexors before you roll up to diminish the lifting effect.

REPETITIONS: One set of ten repetitions.

BREATHING: Breathe out on the roll up, breathe in on the stretch forward, and breathe out on the roll down.

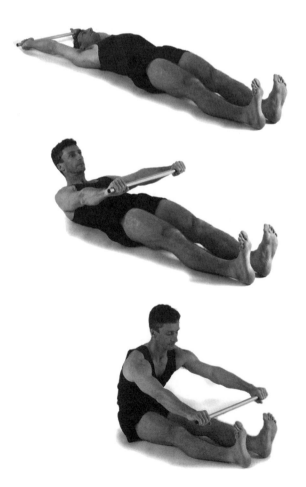

THE PSOAS AND ITS EFFECT ON THE BACK

The psoas and its effect on the back during roll-ups or conventional sit-ups is greatly underestimated. When you rest between repetitions (even for a fraction of a second), the torso will lift off the floor and the hip flexors will engage at the same time, pulling the body up. This is more apparent when the feet are hooked under a strap, as in a gym situation.

Each repetition becomes an individual movement when the head rests for even a fraction of a second. The abdominals then also release for a fraction of a second, and on the next repetition the body lurches forward again. This is because the psoas grips. It therefore controls the movement and lifts the lower lumbar vertebrae, slightly distending the abdominals. This, together with weak abdominals, does not depress the psoas to allow the spine to roll up. The result is a lift of the back.

Instead of completing ten "individual" movements, keep the abdominals and hip flexors connected and try to perform ten connected movements. Think of the set as one movement comprising ten continuous parts.

If the hip flexors are continuously engaged and the abdominals are in a strong B-Line (to assist in depressing the psoas) before the roll-up begins, the chances of a lurch are greatly minimized. Initially, the thighs may feel overworked. However, as the abdominals retain the engram (memory) of the rolling movement, they will supersede any hip flexor strain. When the feet are in a strap to assist in the roll-up, imagine that the strap is a thin thread of cotton and any mild pull of the feet will snap that thread. This will also help to disengage the psoas, even partially, and engage more of the abdominals.

The feet should remain flexed at all times. When they are in a strap that is around the toes, this only engages the thighs even more. Place the strap close to the ankles.

Squeezing the inner thighs may also help slightly to alleviate the hip flexor connection.

NOTES

Exercise 34
THE ROLL-OVER (OR SPINE ROLL)

PREREQUISITES: Two sets of The Hundreds (Exercise 19-1) with low legs, and an absence of neck problems.

PURPOSE: To mobilize and massage the length of the spine and shoulders, and to open the vertebral spaces while flexing the spine. This exercise is similar to the yoga plough.

EXERCISE DESCRIPTION:

Starting Position: Lie on your back on the floor, with the legs vertical, feet pointed and turned out. Squeeze the back of the knees, hands by your sides, palms down. Do the B-Line.

a) Breathe out as you draw the thighs to the rib cage (legs still straight), folding from the hips, and continue rolling over smoothly. Elongate the knees to your nose until the feet touch the floor, if you can. Roll over only onto the top of the shoulders, lengthening the neck. Maintain the B-Line.

b) Breathe in as you turn the legs in and open them to just past shoulder-width apart. Flex the feet.

c) Breathe out as you roll the spine one vertebra at a time, imprinting it back onto the mat until the legs are back in the starting position.

KEY POINTS: Imagine you have heavy ankle weights on your ankles, and keep your knees stretched straight. This will keep the legs closer to the body and increase the stretch of the spine and hamstrings. Use light to medium ankle weights if this helps. On the way back to the floor, scrape your thighs along your chest, extending through the heels to a point above your head and horizontal to the floor. Move over your head smoothly, without using momentum; use only the strength from your abdominals. Keep the thighs close to your chest on the roll-over (draw the hips to the ribs) and on the roll down (lengthen the hips away from the ribs). Concentrate on keeping the stomach hollow. Keep the shoulders relaxed, putting hardly any pressure into the arms or hands.

CARE: Do not roll onto the neck; keep the neck elongated at all times. If you can comfortably touch the floor above the head with your feet, you can obtain more stretch in the hamstrings and spine by flexing the feet with the legs parallel, anchoring the toes into the floor, and pressing into the heels. Elongate the stomach on the roll down to prevent the neck arching and the shoulders lifting.

REPETITIONS: Five repetitions as just described and five in the reverse direction: Roll over with the legs apart, feet flexed and parallel. Roll down with the legs together and turned out, feet pointed.

ADVANCED VERSION: Extend the arms above the head, with the palms up, so you are not using the arms and can more effectively use the abdominals; keep the elbows and wrists pressed into the floor. On the roll down, press the elbows and shoulders into the mat; slowly release the abdominals (do not keep them contracted). Imagine they are pressing and releasing each vertebra into the mat. This will prevent the head and shoulders from lifting off the mat.

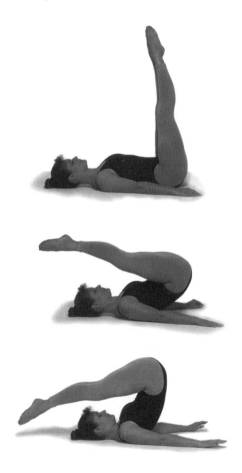

Exercise 35
SINGLE LEG CIRCLES

PREREQUISITE: Single Leg Circles 1 (Exercise 22).

PURPOSE: To isolate the adductor muscle and to mobilize the hip joint.

EXERCISE DESCRIPTION:

Starting Position: Lie on the floor with both legs bent. Extend the arms out to the sides on the floor, palms up. Do the B-Line. Raise the right leg to the ceiling, point the foot, and turn out the leg. Press the left buttock into the mat.

a) As you make a counterclockwise circle, breathe out as you take the leg across the body to the left and then lower the leg to the floor, allowing the abdominals to stretch. Extend through the toes while making a large circle out to the far right.

b) Breathe in as you raise the leg to the vertical position, and do the B-Line. The circle is a rapid movement as the leg is lowered and extended to the side. It is a slower movement as the leg is raised and crosses the body.

Eventually, attempt to make the circle as close to the floor as possible without the opposite hip moving at all.

KEY POINTS: Feel the inner thigh (adductor) muscle making the circle. Keep the circle high and small to start. Do not allow the leg to lower too far if the back arches. Press the fingers of the right hand into the right adductor to feel the connection for this muscle. Keep the left foot in the tripod position.

CARE: Do not push the arms onto the floor.

REPETITIONS: Six circles in one direction, then change legs. Repeat the circles in the other direction.

ADVANCED: Extend the bent leg onto the floor, with the foot flexed.

NOTES

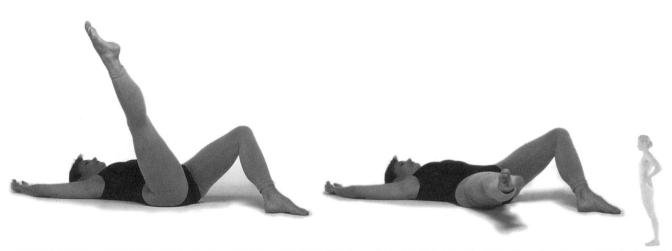

Exercise 36
DOUBLE LEG STRETCH 2: LOWERING AND RAISING

PREREQUISITES: Preparation for the Hundreds (Exercise 17), Double Leg Stretch: Basic (Exercise 21), The Hundreds: Alternating Legs (Exercise 31), and Coordination (Exercise 32).

PURPOSE: To gain abdominal strength and control when moving the lower limbs, as well as to increase breathing control and shoulder mobility.

EXERCISE DESCRIPTION:

Starting Position: Complete the starting position of the basic Double Leg Stretch (Exercise 21), this time keeping the legs just past the vertical position, away from the body. Complete the arm circle.

a) Hold this position and take a deep breath in.

b) Breathe out as you lower the legs as low as you can without lifting the back, keeping the feet flexed and turned out, and squeezing the inner thighs (Figure i).

c) Do the B-Line harder and breathe in as you raise the legs back to the vertical position, still squeezing the inner thighs.

d) Breathe out as you extend the hands to the ceiling and continue, on the same breath, to complete a second circle with the arms (Figure ii).

e) Breathe in and return to the starting position (Figure iii).

KEY POINTS: When lowering the legs, press through the heels. Keep the shoulder blades just off the floor at all times. It is important not to allow the head and shoulders to lower as the legs lower. This may arch the back, which may then strain when lifting the legs. You should feel as if the abdominals are flattening and lengthening to allow the legs to lower. When raising the legs, do the B-Line first and feel the hips drawing to the rib cage. Feel as if the action of the abdominals contracting is what raises the legs into the air.

CARE: If the exercise is too challenging at first, return to the resting position after the legs have been raised—do not complete the second circle. If, after several repetitions, the back begins to arch, do not lower the legs too far.

REPETITIONS: One set of ten, with half a second of rest between each repetition.

BREATHING: Breathe out as you contract forward. Breathe in while moving the arms to the vertical position. Breathe out as you move the arms around in a big circle. Breathe in as you hold the position with the hands by the sides. Breathe out as you lower the legs. Breathe in as you raise the legs. Breathe out during the second full circle (optional). Breathe in as you rest for half a second.

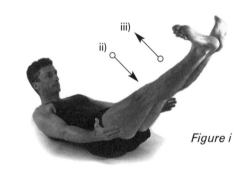

Figure i

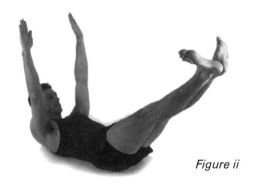

Figure ii

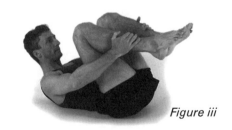

Figure iii

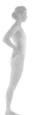

VARIATION TO MAKE THE ABDOMINALS WORK HARDER

PREREQUISITE: Double Leg Stretch 2 (Exercise 36).

Follow all the instructions for the Double Leg Stretch, and then continue as described in the instructions that follow.

ARMS TO CEILING: After completing the first circle,

    a) Breathe in as you raise your arms to the vertical position.

    b) Breathe out as you lower the legs and continue as before (Figure i).

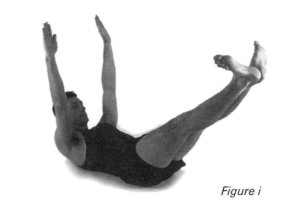

Figure i

ARMS TO EARS: After completing the first circle,

    a) Breathe in as you raise your arms past the vertical position so that they are in line with your ears.

    b) Breathe out as you lower the legs and continue as before (Figure ii).

EXPANSION: After completing the first circle,

    a) Breathe in as you raise the arms vertically.

    b) Breathe out as you lower the right leg and extend the right arm to the right ear.

    c) Breathe in as you raise the leg and arm.

    d) Breathe out as you repeat with the other arm and leg. Continue as before (Figure iii).

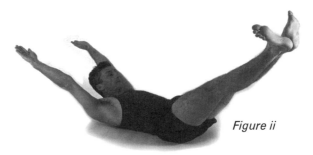

Figure ii

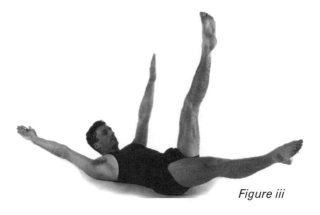

Figure iii

Exercise 37
ROLLING

PREREQUISITES: The Roll-Up (Exercise 33), The Perfect Abdominal Curl (Exercise 25).

PURPOSE: To stretch and mobilize the spine.

EXERCISE DESCRIPTION:

Starting Position: Sit on the floor on a mat with your heels drawn to your tailbone, forehead resting between your knees, which should be slightly apart. Cross your right ankle over your left, and clasp your hands on your top ankle, holding tight. Do the B-Line.

a) Sink into your hips and round your back. At the same time, breathe out as you roll smoothly onto your spine up to your shoulder blades, keeping your heels to the tailbone, and lengthen your neck.

b) Breathe in as you pull your hands sharply to the floor to initiate the movement back to the upright position. Balance on your tailbone with the toes lightly touching the floor.

KEY POINTS: Keep the heels close to the tailbone. Roll only onto the shoulders, not onto the neck. Sink into the hips to start the movement; this will help curl the tailbone to start the smooth roll. You may find that you will roll to one side of the mat at first, but this will become less likely as you perform more sets and gain better balance.

CARE: If the back has any "flat spots" at all, stop. Flat spots are sections of the spine that do not roll smoothly, making you spend more effort on lifting the body off the ground than on rolling smoothly.

REPETITIONS: One set of ten rolls.

NOTES

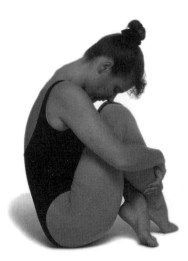

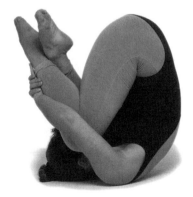

SINGLE LEG STRETCH WITH ROTATION: CRISS-CROSS

PREREQUISITES: The Perfect Abdominal Curl (Exercise 25), Single Leg Stretch (Exercise 20).

PURPOSE: To strengthen the obliques.

EXERCISE DESCRIPTION:

In essence, this exercise is the same as the Perfect Abdominal Curls and Single Leg Stretch combined.

Starting Position: Lying on the floor, contract forward with the hands behind the head and the elbows open.

a) Breathe out and curl the body forward, drawing the right armpit toward the left knee, drawing the knee toward the left shoulder. Extend the right leg, pointed and turned out, as low to the floor as possible without the back lifting. Scoop the stomach.

b) Breathing in, change legs and release the torso until the shoulder blades almost touch the floor.

Repeat on the other side.

KEY POINTS: Keep the shoulder blades off the floor at all times. Keep the elbows open. Turn the head and shoulders and look to the side for maximum rotation of the torso (where the eyes go, the body follows). Keep the hips still, planted into the mat. Maintain the B-Line at all times. Be sure to extend the legs in line with the hip, not out to the sides.

CARE: Keep the elbows open so there is no strain on the neck. Keep the chin off the chest, eyes forward except when turning. When turning to the side, keep both shoulders off the floor.

REPETITIONS: One set of ten on each side.

NOTES

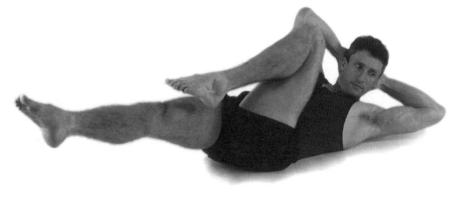

Exercise 39
STOMACH STRETCH: ALTERNATING ARMS AND LEGS

PREREQUISITE: Stomach Stretch (Exercise 24).

PURPOSE: To strengthen the back muscles.

EXERCISE DESCRIPTION:

Starting Position: Lie on the stomach with the arms and legs extended shoulder-width apart. Place a small, flat cushion between the hips and the ribs to help support the B-Line. Rest the forehead on the floor or on a cushion. Point and turn out the legs.

a) Maintaining the B-Line and breathing out, lift and lengthen the opposite arm and leg less than 2 inches off the floor. Pinch the buttocks, but do not grip. At the same time, imagine that your abdominals are like a greyhound's stomach.

b) Keeping the buttocks pinched, breathe in as you slowly lower the arm and leg and switch to the other arm and leg.

KEY POINTS: Maintain the B-Line to prevent the back from arching. Allow the movement to flow smoothly. Keep the muscles of the arm and leg, which are in contact with the floor, "holding" (not fully rested). Relax the neck, drawing the shoulder blades to the hips. Lengthen through the tips of the fingers and toes.

CARE: If you feel any twinges in the back, draw the stomach in harder. If this is of no assistance, stop the exercise after only a few repetitions. Lengthen the neck. If your head drops below the level of the shoulders, place the forehead on a higher cushion, so that the neck is not arching.

REPETITIONS: Six to ten lifts on each side.

NOTES

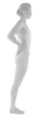

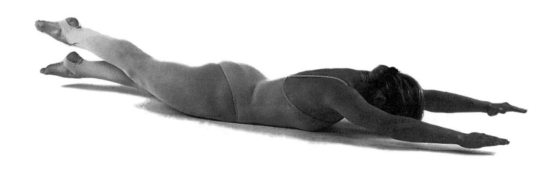

Exercise 40
SINGLE LEG KICK

PREREQUISITES: The Hundreds: Intermediate (Exercise 19-1) and a strong back.

PURPOSE: To firm the hamstrings and buttocks, strengthen the abdominals in an elongated position, and stretch the front of the thighs.

EXERCISE DESCRIPTION:

Starting Position: Lie on your stomach on the floor, legs extended, toes pointed.

a) Do the B-Line and rise up onto your elbows, keeping them directly below your shoulders, palms down and pressed into the mat. Lengthen through the crown of the head without arching your neck. Keep the hips pressed into the mat and lift your chest as high as you can, stretching the abdominals, but maintain the B-Line to support the back. Stretch through the toes, squeeze the buttocks firmly, and lift the feet just off the ground.

b) Breathe out as you rapidly kick your right foot to your buttock twice. On the second kick, lower the foot only halfway to the floor and then kick to the buttock with the foot flexed.

c) Point the foot and breathe in as you lower the leg to the floor.

d) Change legs.

KEY POINTS: If the hips lift off the floor and the back feels tight, extend the elbows farther in front of you, so that your back is longer. Make sure the hipbones stay on the floor. Keep the rib cage lengthened away from the hips. Breathe out sharply and quickly for each kick.

CARE: If you feel the back starting to take any pressure, do the B-Line more firmly. If the pressure continues, stop the exercise. Keep the back of the neck in a long curve in line with the upper part of the back. Use the pressure of the palms to stabilize yourself, keeping the fingers extended.

REPETITIONS: One set of five kicks on each leg, alternating legs.

BREATHING: Breathe out on the double kick. Breathe in when lowering the leg.

NOTES

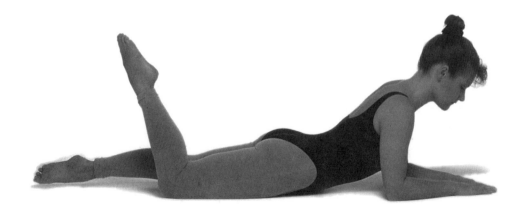

Exercise 41
DOUBLE LEG KICK

PREREQUISITE: Single Leg Kick (Exercise 40).

PURPOSE: To firm the buttocks and hamstrings, strengthen the back, and open the chest.

EXERCISE DESCRIPTION:

Starting Position: Lie on your stomach with your head turned to the right. Keep the legs straight, feet pointed. Hold one hand with the other, behind your back as high up toward the shoulder blades as you can, with the elbows touching the floor. Do the B-Line and "zip" up the stomach (Figure i).

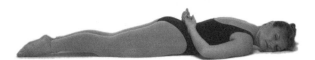

Figure i

a) Breathe out as you rapidly kick your feet together to your buttocks three times (Figure ii).

b) Breathe in as you then stretch the legs away from the body as high as you can. At the same time, stretch your hands toward your feet, still holding them together.

c) Lift your chest off the floor as high as possible without arching your neck, looking toward the ceiling (Figure iii).

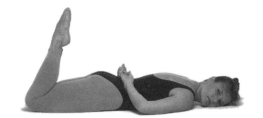

Figure ii

d) Breathe in as you return to the starting position with your head turned in the other direction.

KEY POINTS: Press the shoulder blades to the hips and keep the neck long. As you lift the chest off the ground, flatten the ribs in a smooth line to the abdominals. Squeeze the buttocks firmly throughout the routine.

CARE: Reduce the intensity or lift of the movement if you feel tightness in the shoulders, neck, or lower back.

REPETITIONS: One set of ten kicks, alternating the direction of the head each time.

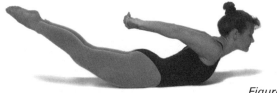

Figure iii

BREATHING: Breathe out as you kick three times, breathe in as you lift and lengthen, and breathe out as you lower the torso and repeat the kicks.

Exercise 42
SWAN DIVE 1
(ROCKING PRESS-UP 1)

PREREQUISITES: Thigh Stretch 3: Kneeling (Exercise 13), the Perfect Abdominal Curl (Exercise 25), Stomach Stretch: Alternating Arms and Legs (Exercise 39).

PURPOSE: To strengthen the back and increase back control.

EXERCISE DESCRIPTION:

Starting Position: Lie on the stomach in the press-up position, hands close to the shoulders, fingers forward. Lengthen through your toes with your legs in a comfortable position (shoulder distance apart). Do the B-Line and keep the buttocks tight, but not gripping.

a) Raise the legs slightly off the ground and, breathing out, straighten your arms as you raise your chest off the mat, letting your thighs contact the mat. Lengthen the head high and back, without feeling any pressure along the spine (Figure i). Lock your body into this position.

b) Breathing in, bend the arms and rock forward. The legs should rise into the air. Reaching the toes to the ceiling, roll as far forward onto your breastbone as possible (Figure ii).

c) Immediately rock back into the straight-arm position (Figure i).

KEY POINTS: If this movement is uncomfortable in the hip area, place a cushion under the hips. Keep the movement smooth at all times, with rhythmic breathing.

CARE: Keep lengthening through the crown of the head and through the point of the toes. Reverse the breathing if it is more comfortable, but maintain the B-Line. Keep the shoulder blades pressed to the hips.

REPETITIONS: Three to eight repetitions.

NOTES

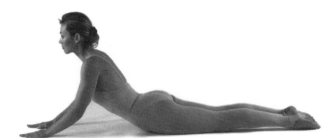

Figure i

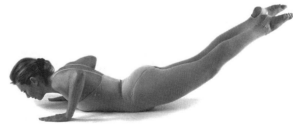

Figure ii

Exercise 42-1
SWAN DIVE 2
(ROCKING PRESS-UP 2)

NOTES

The movement is the same as that in Exercise 42.

a) After straightening the arms, in a rapid movement lift them up off the floor in line with your ears (Figure i).

b) Extend your arms forward with the palms facing down, which will make your body rock forward.

c) Breathing out, rock as far forward onto your breastbone as possible before rocking back as high as you can, breathing in (Figure ii).

Continue rocking, keeping the movement as smooth as possible.

Complete three to eight repetitions. Follow all the other instructions as for Exercise 42.

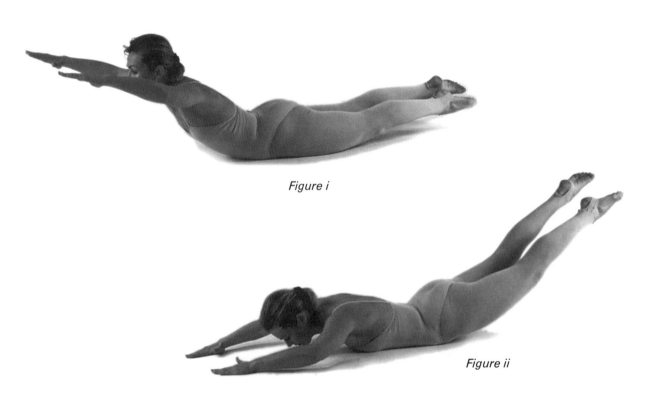

Figure i

Figure ii

Exercise 43
SWIMMING

PREREQUISITES: The Hundreds: Intermediate (Exercise 19-1), Stomach Stretch: Alternating Arms and Legs (Exercise 39).

PURPOSE: To strengthen the back muscles and mobilize the hips and shoulders.

EXERCISE DESCRIPTION:

Starting Position: Lie on the floor with the arms and legs extended, feet slightly apart.

a) Do the B-Line, lightly tighten the buttocks, and lift the arms, chest, and legs 6 inches off the floor. Lengthen through the tips of the fingers and toes, keeping the shoulders and pelvis square. Move the shoulder blades to the hips.

b) From this starting position, raise the right arm and left leg 4 inches higher. Breathe out as you quickly alternate the arms and legs for five beats.

c) Breathe in for five beats.

KEY POINTS: Maintain the B-Line. Keep the shoulders relaxed, shoulder blades to hips. Extend the arms and legs through the fingertips and toes.

CARE: Keep the legs to a height where the abdominals are pulled away from the floor to prevent the back from taking over.

REPETITIONS: One set of ten breaths in and out.

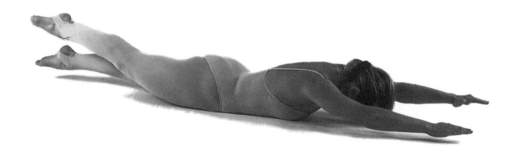

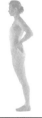

Exercise 44
SPINE ROTATION (SPINE TWIST)

PREREQUISITES: The Start Stretches (Exercises 3 to 6a).

PURPOSE: To provide mobility in the spine in rotation, and to focus on lifting out of the hips.

EXERCISE DESCRIPTION:

Starting Position: Sit upright on your sit bones on a mat, with your legs straight in front of you, and press through the heels, keeping them together. Without hunching the shoulders, raise your arms to shoulder height, palms down, stretching through the fingertips; lift the ribs away from the hips and stretch the crown of your head to the ceiling (Figure i).

    a) Do the B-Line and breathe out deeply as you rotate the body to the right as far as you can. Initiate the movement from the rib cage and, flattening the ribs as you rotate, maintain the erect posture. Imagine you are turning on the base of your spine (Figure ii).

    b) When you have rotated as far as you can, hold the position for half a second (keeping the ribs flat and the posture erect), and breathe out more as you rotate a little farther, this time turning the right shoulder blade as far back as possible.

    c) Breathe in as you return to the starting position, and, without stopping, smoothly flow into a rotation in the other direction.

KEY POINTS: Keep lifted out of the hips. Keep the shoulder blades pressed to the hips at all times. Turn the head with the shoulders and feel the movement loosening the rib cage area. Do not allow the hips to move.

CARE: Do only the number of repetitions that are comfortable for the neck and shoulders. Perform the movement slowly without much rotation at first, and, as you warm up, go faster, increasing the rotation each time.

REPETITIONS: Try to do ten.

NOTES

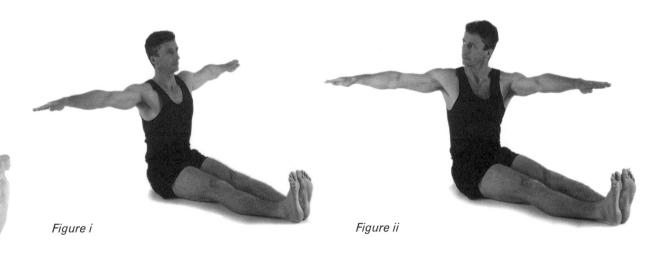

Figure i

Figure ii

Exercise 45
SPINE STRETCH

PREREQUISITES: The Start Stretches (Exercises 3 to 6a), hamstrings and thighs (Exercises 9-1 to 13).

PURPOSE: To stretch the spine and the hamstrings.

EXERCISE DESCRIPTION:

Starting Position: Sit upright on the sit bones with the legs slightly wider apart than shoulder distance, feet flexed, knees pressed to the floor. Lift the arms to the ceiling and lift the ribs vertically from the hips, with the shoulder blades to the hips.

a) Breathe out as you curl the chin down to the rib cage, then move the nose to the B-Line. Extend the arms in front of you as far forward as possible without hunching the shoulders, keeping the nose toward the B-Line (Figure i).

b) Breathe in and hold the position.

c) Breathing out, lengthen the spine forward as far as possible (Figure ii).

d) Hold the stretch, breathing in.

e) Breathe out as you curl the spine back to the upright position, still reaching through the fingertips as far forward as possible.

KEY POINTS: If you feel any discomfort in the back of the knees, bend them slightly. Keep the shoulder blades pressed to the hips. Curl on the return to the upright position. Start by doing the B-Line, then stack the vertebrae one at a time on top of each other, lifting the ribs from the hips, keeping the nose to the B-Line until the very end. Then lift the head upright. Focus on deep breathing at all times.

CARE: Do not force the movement. As you complete more of these, you will gradually become looser.

REPETITIONS: One set of ten stretches.

BREATHING: Breathe out on curling the nose to the B-Line. Breathe in as you hold the position. Breathe out as you stretch forward. Breathe in as you hold, and breathe out on the return to the upright position.

NOTES

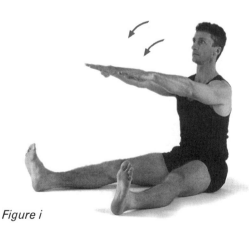

Figure i

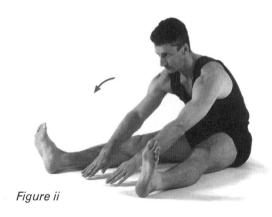

Figure ii

Exercise 46
OPEN LEG ROCKER

PREREQUISITES: The Start Stretches (Exercises 3 to 6a), Hamstring Stretches (Exercises 9-1 to 10), The Perfect Abdominal Curl (Exercise 25), The Roll-Over (or Spine Roll) (Exercise 34).

PURPOSE: To improve balance.

EXERCISE DESCRIPTION:

Starting Position: Sit tall on the floor with your knees bent open, toes pointed and close to your tailbone, hands on the ankles inside the open knees (Figure i).

a) Do the B-Line and, balancing on your tailbone, straighten your legs into the air to form a V. Keep the arms straight (Figure ii).

b) Curve your back into a C shape by sinking into your hips (with control), and breathe out as you smoothly roll along your spine to the top of your shoulders (Figure iii).

c) Breathe in as you roll back to the upright position, sitting tall, chin up, spine long. Repeat the exercise from the starting position.

KEY POINTS: A great deal of balance and abdominal control is required for this exercise. When the legs are extended into the air, try to align the toes with the top of your head. Keep the ribs to the hips on the roll-over and the roll-up. Press the abdominals in the direction of the hips as hard as possible for both movements. On the roll-up, flatten the ribs as you sit in the upright position as if you had a rod through your spine from the tailbone to the crown of your head.

CARE: Roll over only onto the top of the shoulders, keeping your chin to your rib cage. If you feel unbalanced as you roll into the upright position, bend the knees slightly to gain more control over the movement. Roll smoothly through the spine—there should be no flat spots.

Beginner's Hint: If you are unable to gain control when doing this movement, try the following:

From the starting position, try to straighten the legs open, then breathe out as you close the legs together, trying to extend the lower back. Keeping your balance, breathe in as you open the legs, sitting taller, and flatten the rib cage. Breathe out as you bend the knees back to the starting position. Repeat six to ten times.

REPETITIONS: One set of six.

BREATHING: Breathe in as you extend the legs, breathe out as you roll back, and breathe in as you roll upright.

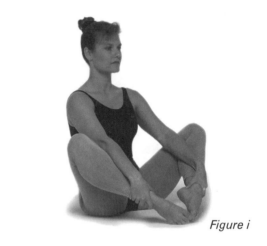

Figure i

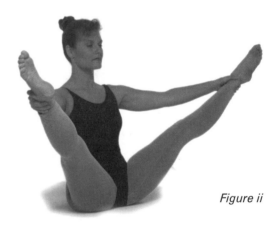

Figure ii

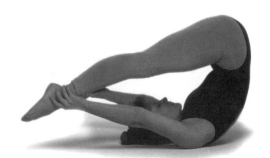

Figure iii

Exercise 47
CORKSCREW: BASIC

PREREQUISITE: The Hundreds: Alternating Legs (Exercise 31).

PURPOSE: To increase oblique and abdominal strength, as well as hip and lower back mobility.

EXERCISE DESCRIPTION:

Starting Position: Lie on the floor, with the arms by the sides, palms down. Extend both legs vertically into the air, feet pointed and turned out, and squeeze the back of the knees together.

a) Do the B-Line and breathe out as both legs lower out to the right side and away from the body into a circle (see Figure).

b) Breathe in as the legs return to the vertical position.

c) Do the B-Line and breathe out as the legs then reverse direction and go to the left. Repeat the exercise, changing directions each time.

Because of the continual change of direction, the obliques and abdominals are required to change their direction of control. This constant redirection of the muscle provides a greater challenge than doing ten circles in the one direction.

KEY POINTS: As the legs lower away from the body, lengthen and flatten the abdominals to prevent the back from arching. Imagine that the movement is being performed from the inner thighs near the groin: this will give you more control. Do not press on the arms.

CARE: Start with small corkscrews, without moving the hips off the floor; then, as you gain more confidence and control, make the corkscrews bigger.

REPETITIONS: One set of six to ten in each direction.

Exercise 47-1:
CORKSCREW 1: INTERMEDIATE

This exercise is similar in all aspects to the basic Corkscrew, except the circle is bigger.

EXERCISE DESCRIPTION: Make the circle bigger to work the abdominals more. As this becomes easier, take the arms out away from the body, keeping the palms up. If the palms are down, there is more tendency to push the hands on the floor to maintain control, rather than using the abdominals; this would also strain the neck and shoulders. As you become more proficient with this version, keep extending the arms above shoulder height on the floor and keep the circle close to the floor. (Do not allow the shoulders to lift off the floor.) This is abdominal control at its best.

NOTES

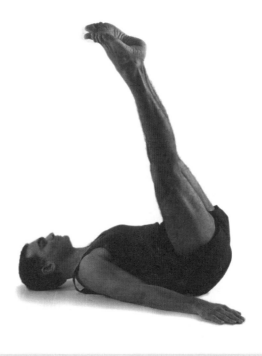

Exercise 47-2
CORKSCREW 2: ADVANCED

PREREQUISITES: Corkscrew: Basic (Exercise 47), The Roll-Over (or Spine Roll) (Exercise 34).

PURPOSE: To strengthen the abdominals, obliques, and spine, and to mobilize the spine and hips.

EXERCISE DESCRIPTION:

Starting Position: Lie flat on your back on the floor, with the legs vertical and turned out, and the feet pointed. Squeeze the back of the knees and keep your arms by your sides, palms down (Figure i).

a) Breathe out and roll over onto the shoulders to the roll-over position, as in Exercise 34 (Figure ii).

b) Hold the position for the breath in.

c) Breathe out as you take the legs to the right side of the body, rolling the hips to the left (Figure iii). Roll onto the right side of the body, lowering the legs into a circle.

d) Breathe in as you roll back up onto the left side of the body into the roll-over position.

e) Breathe out as you now reverse the movement, rolling onto the left side of the body.

KEY POINTS: The farther over into the roll-over you are, the better. However, remain on the top of the shoulders only. The bigger the circle (out to the sides and down to the floor), the more challenging the exercise. Keep the movement fluid and the roll smooth. Try to place the least amount of pressure possible on the hands. Keep the shoulders relaxed, and use the abdominals. Keep the legs turned out, stretching through the toes. Maintain the B-Line at all times!

CARE: If the back arches too much, or the shoulders do most of the work, stop the exercise. Keep the breathing smooth and deep—do not hold your breath. Keep the back of the neck long and pressed into the mat. Keep the shoulder blades pressed to the hips.

REPETITIONS: Up to five complete movements (one complete corkscrew is a roll onto the side in each direction).

BREATHING: Breathe out as you roll the back to the floor and stretch the legs away. Breathe in as you roll onto the shoulders with the legs above the head.

Note: It may be a good idea to review the notes on breathing at this point. See "General Breathing Rules" in Chapter 2.

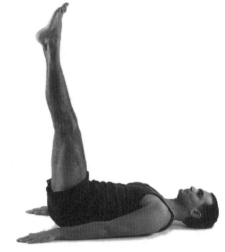

Figure i

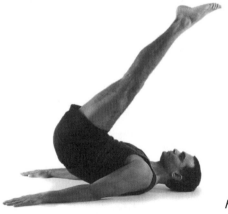

Figure ii

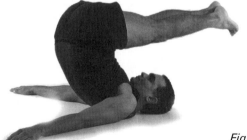

Figure iii

PREREQUISITE: Spine Stretch (Exercise 45).

PURPOSE: To provide basic rotation of the spine, concentrating on the rib cage.

EXERCISE DESCRIPTION:

Starting Position: Sit upright on the floor as if there were a rod through your spine. Extend the arms out to the sides, parallel to the floor, reaching through the fingertips, as if a pole were extended from one fingertip, through the shoulders, to the other fingertip (Figure i).

 a) Breathe out as you rotate the torso to the right by turning the rib cage and at the same time reaching forward with the left hand toward the outside of the right foot (Figure ii).

 b) Keep breathing out as you imitate a sawing action with the edge of the right hand halfway up the outside edge of the foot for two short strokes. Taking two sharper breaths out for each of the sawing movements will help you to stretch farther.

 c) Breathe in as you return to the upright position by rolling the rib cage back using the oblique muscles.

 d) Stretch to one side, then return to the upright position. Stretch to the other side with a continuous, flowing movement, then return again to the upright position.

KEY POINTS: As you reach forward to "saw off" the foot, rotate the torso as if you were trying to turn your chest toward the ceiling. Lengthen through the crown of the head. Press both buttocks firmly into the floor at all times. Keep the feet flexed. Do not rest the head on the shoulder when rotating the torso.

CARE: If you cannot reach the foot, do not force the stretch. It is more important to control the rotation from the anterior part of the torso. Rotate and reach only as far as is comfortable. For some of you, this may be only 50 percent of what is shown in the photograph. This is fine: progress gradually from the point you find comfortable.

REPETITIONS: Up to ten stretches to each side, alternating sides.

BREATHING: Breathe out as you rotate and reach, and breathe out in two further short breaths on the saw. Breathe in and rotate back to the upright position.

NOTES

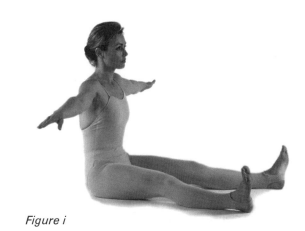

Figure i

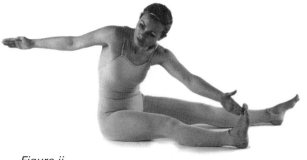

Figure ii

Exercise 49
SIDE KICK 1

PREREQUISITES: The Start Stretches (Exercises 3 to 6a), The Hundreds: Alternating Legs (Exercise 31).

PURPOSE: To mobilize the hips, stretch the hamstrings, and strengthen the lower back.

EXERCISE DESCRIPTION:

Starting Position: Lie on the floor on your right side, balancing on your right hip, with your head resting on your right arm, elbow in line with the body, and left hand palm-down on the mat by your waist.

a) Keeping your legs straight, bring them slightly forward, with both feet flexed and lengthened through the heels. Press the right toes into the floor. Lift the left leg slightly to hip level, keep the foot flexed, and do the B-Line (Figure i).

b) Take a deep breath in as you kick the left leg forward as far as you can, pressing through the heel. Keep the spine straight (Figure ii).

c) At the end of the kick, do a further, smaller kick, inhaling an extra breath to expand the lungs more.

d) Point your foot and breathe out as you kick your leg back in a sweeping motion, stretching through the top of the thigh, and do the B-Line harder (Figure iii). Flatten the rib cage and keep the back as straight as you can.

e) Flex the foot and press through the heel for the next kick forward.

Repeat on the other side.

KEY POINTS: Stabilize your center and, as if your hip were the center of a circle, lengthen through the heel and toe, reaching past the outer rim of the circle. Keep the shoulders stable and the chin lifted. Lengthen through the crown of the head. To keep the top hip directly above the bottom one, create a small gap between the waist and the floor.

CARE: If you feel any strain in the back, discontinue the exercise. If you feel the hipbone on the mat, place a flat cushion under the hip.

REPETITIONS: Ten kicks on each side.

BREATHING: Breathe in as you kick forward, and take an extra breath in at the stretch. Breathe out as you kick back.

NOTES

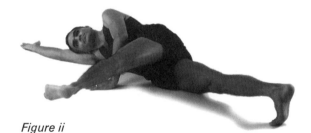

Figure i

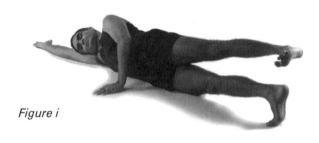

Figure ii

Figure iii

Exercise 50-1
SIDE LEG LIFTS

PREREQUISITE: The Hundreds: Alternating Legs (Exercise 31).

PURPOSE: To strengthen the side muscles of the waist (quadratus lumborum), the obliques, and the muscles of the outside of the thigh (tensor fascia lata).

EXERCISE DESCRIPTION:

Starting Position: Lie on your left side with your head resting on your left arm, elbow in line with the body. Place the right hand lightly on the floor by the waist. Keep the legs parallel, slightly in front of the body, with the toes pointed. There should be a small gap between the left waistband and the floor. Tuck the pelvis posteriorly to assist in maintaining a flatter back.

a) Do the B-Line and breathe out as you lift both legs as high as you can without leaning the hips backward.

b) Breathe in as you lower the legs slowly until they almost touch the floor. Repeat the exercise.

KEY POINTS: Maintain the gap between the waistband and the floor. Sigh deeply on the breath out.

For beginners, to prevent the hips from rolling back, keep your back flat against a wall without leaning against it.

CARE: If there is an arch in the back, flatten it by connecting the lower abdominals more with the posterior tuck. If there is still an arch, keep both legs forward of the straight line of the body, so the back does not excessively engage. Keep the supporting hand relaxed—do not use it to push on the floor, as this will hunch the shoulder. Place a thin cushion between the thighs and squeeze as you lift for more control and tone of the adductor muscles. If you feel pressure on the bottom hip as you lift the legs, place a flat cushion under the hip.

REPETITIONS: Ten lifts, then change and repeat on the other side.

ADVANCED: Raise your left hand behind your head, with the elbow behind your ear and to the ceiling. Greater balance is required for this version.

Exercise 50-2:
SIDE LEG KICK

Lie in the same starting position as in the Side Leg Lifts (Exercise 50-1).

a) Turn out the top leg so the kneecap is facing the ceiling, and point the foot.

b) Do the B-Line and breathe in as you kick up to the ceiling. Do not lean back.

c) Flex the foot and breathe out as you press through the heel, lowering back to the other foot. Repeat ten times, then change sides.

NOTES

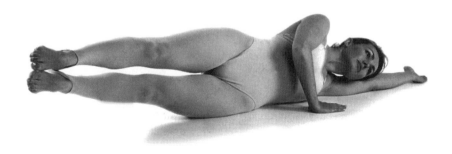

Exercise 51
PELVIC CURL

PREREQUISITE: None.

PURPOSE: To help open and mobilize the lower back, and to connect the lower abdominals.

EXERCISE DESCRIPTION: This exercise is best done with the legs on a chair.

Starting Position: Lie on your back with your feet on a chair, hip-distance apart. The thigh bone should be at a 90-degree angle to the floor. If the feet are too close to the buttocks, more pressure will be applied to the lower back.

a) With the palms facing up by your sides, do the B-Line and, breathing out, draw the hipbones to the rib cage and continue to do so until the pelvis tilts off the floor about 2 to 4 inches.

b) Breathing in, slowly release the hips down to the floor. Maintain abdominal control throughout the movement.

KEY POINTS: It may help to gently press the fingers of one hand into the lower abdominals to feel the connection of the abdominal muscles.

CARE: Do not press on the arms or feet to achieve this movement. Do not tense the shoulders, lengthening the neck. Do not press on the heels. Do not allow the back to arch at any time.

REPETITIONS: Two sets of ten repetitions.

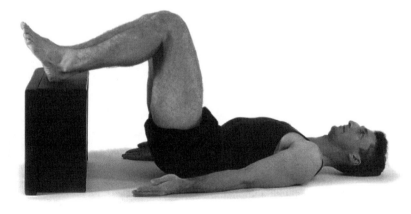

Exercise 52
PELVIC LIFT

PREREQUISITE & PURPOSE: Same as for the Pelvic Curl (Exercise 51). This exercise will also strengthen and tighten the buttocks.

EXERCISE DESCRIPTION: The Pelvic Lift starts in the same position as the Pelvic Curl, except lifting higher.

a) After you have achieved the curl, continue breathing out and peel the spine off the floor until the hips are raised off the floor. Do not arch the lower back; you should feel no pressure in the spine. Control all the work from the abdominals.

b) Breathe in and imprint the spine one vertebra at a time when releasing the position.

KEY POINTS: Same as for the Pelvic Curl.

CARE: Do not place any pressure on the heels. The knees should be hip-distance apart and at a right angle above the navel when in the resting position. Remember to peel the spine off the floor and to imprint it back on the floor. Do not peel the spine off any higher than is comfortable, and do not arch the back.

REPETITIONS: One set of ten repetitions.

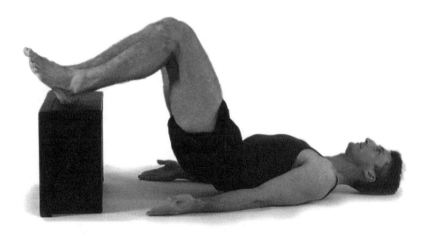

Exercise 53-1
TEASER 1: BASIC

PREREQUISITES: The Hundreds: Alternating Legs (Exercise 31), The Perfect Abdominal Curl (Exercise 25), The Roll-Over (or Spine Roll) (Exercise 34).

PURPOSE: To strengthen the abdominals through a continuous movement.

EXERCISE DESCRIPTION:

Starting Position: Lie on your back with your knees bent, arms above the head on the floor. Extend one leg into the air, keeping both knees at the same level (Figure i).

a) Extend your hands, shoulder-distance apart, in a line just above the B-Line, and breathe out as you roll your spine off the mat in a long curve like the arch of a bow, keeping the neck long.

b) As you come up to the highest point, without putting any pressure on the feet, extend the fingers farther to the line above the toes. Avoid rounding the shoulders.

c) Breathe in and straighten the back, opening the chest; lift the ribs from the hips, and sit tall on the sit bones (Figure ii).

d) Breathe out as you lower yourself back to the mat, starting with a very small posterior pelvic tuck (or sinking into the hips), keeping the back extended like the curve of a long bow, moving back to the stretch position.

e) Do not rest. Keep all the muscles engaged and move immediately to the next repetition.

KEY POINTS: Flatten the ribs before the lift, to keep the ribs and upper abdominals in a flat line throughout the movement. Keep the shoulder blades pressed to the hips, and lengthen the neck. Lift tall out of the hips as if you were trying to extend the lower back. Try to achieve the "greyhound's stomach" even while extending the back—this is a challenge!

CARE: If you feel the tops of the thighs overworking, do fewer repetitions or do some Thigh Stretches (Exercise 11 to 13) before continuing.

REPETITIONS: Up to eight repetitions.

BREATHING: Breathe out on the torso lift, and breathe in as you lower back to the floor.

ADVANCED: Lie on your back with both feet resting lightly on a box or high chair, legs parallel and extended at approximately a 45-degree angle, feet softly pointed. Keep your arms above the head on the floor. Continue as in section a), above.

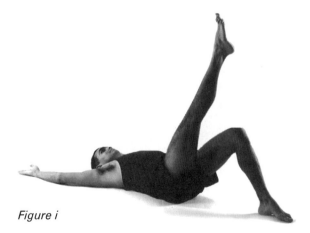

Figure i

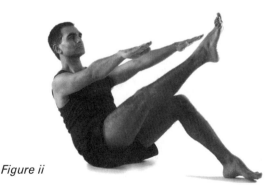

Figure ii

Exercise 53-2
TEASER 2

PREREQUISITE: Teaser 1: Basic (Exercise 53-1).

PURPOSE: To increase abdominal strength, hip mobility, and hip flexor control, and to stretch the lower back.

EXERCISE DESCRIPTION:

Starting Position: Sit tall on your sit bones, legs extended parallel, toes pointed. Your arms should be at shoulder level, extended forward.

a) Do the B-Line and breathe in. Lean the torso back at a 45-degree angle as you raise the legs into a V sit-up. Lift the legs level with your head (or as close as you can), balancing on your sit bones. See if you can touch your toes to your fingers, keeping the back straight, the shoulder blades to the hips, and the neck long.

b) Pause for a second, consolidating the strength of the abdominals and the firm lengthening of the torso. Squeeze the inner thighs.

c) Breathe out as you lower the legs, extending through the toes to just off the floor, back to the starting position. Do not rest.

d) Repeat.

KEY POINTS: Keep the shoulders relaxed and the neck in line with the upper back. Keep the ribs flat when the torso extends. Stretch through the crown of the head and through the point of the toes.

CARE & REPETITIONS: Same as for Exercise 53-1.

NOTES

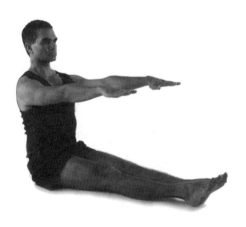
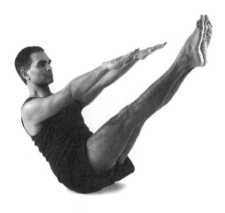

Exercise 53-3
TEASER 3

PREREQUISITE: Teaser 2 (Exercise 53-2).

PURPOSE: To increase balance and control.

EXERCISE DESCRIPTION:

Starting Position: Lie on your back (supine), legs extended parallel, feet pointed. Extend the arms through the fingertips above the head, shoulder-width apart.

a) Do the B-Line and breathe out as you lift the legs, arms, and torso in one movement into a V sit-up position. Balance on your sit bones, reaching for the toes with the fingers. Keep the back as upright as possible (as if there were a rod in your spine). Keep the neck long.

b) Breathe in as you slightly tuck the pelvis, contracting the abdominals. Slowly elongate the torso, legs, and arms back onto the mat at the same time, to the starting position.

ADVANCED: When you have lifted the legs, extend the arms up to the ceiling in line with your ears, shoulder blades to hips. Then continue with section b), above.

KEY POINTS & CARE: Same as for Teaser 1 (Exercise 53-1).

REPETITIONS: Up to ten repetitions.

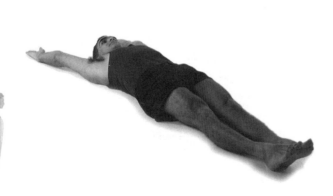

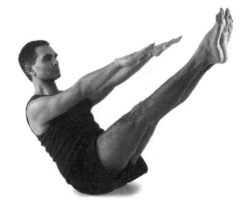

Exercise 54
LEG PULL FRONT

PREREQUISITE: The Hundreds: Alternating Legs (Exercise 31).

PURPOSE: To open the hip joints and strengthen the lower back and shoulders.

EXERCISE DESCRIPTION:

Starting Position: Assume a push-up position: arms locked, fingers pointing forward, and shoulders, hips, and heels in a straight line.

a) Do the B-Line with a slight tuck to help connect the lower abdominals. Keep the neck long in a straight line with the back. Press the heels into the floor as far as you can. Tighten the buttocks.

b) Breathe in as you lift the left leg, with the foot flexed hard, as high as you can to the ceiling (keep the knee joint locked) without allowing the hips to move or the back to arch.

c) Breathe out as you lower the leg to the floor, lengthening farther through the heel. Touch the toe on the mat and repeat on the same leg.

ADVANCED: At the top of the leg lift, do a double kick with an extra breath out. Point the foot as it touches the floor.

KEY POINTS: As you breathe in and extend the leg up, flatten the rib cage and tuck the pelvis. Consciously feel the abdominals tighten and support the entire body. Lengthen through the crown of the head in a straight line through the heels. Maintain the B-Line and keep the abdominals continuously firm. Keep the balance of the toes between the joints of the big toe and the second toe.

CARE: Keep the elbows lengthened and locked. Do not hyperextend, as this may cause a strain at the elbow joint.

REPETITIONS: One set of five repetitions on each leg.

BREATHING: Breathe in as you lift the leg. Breathe out as you lower the leg.

NOTES

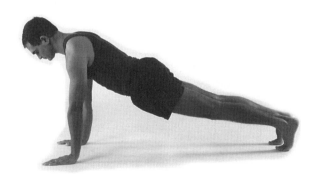
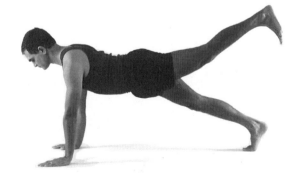

Exercise 55
LEG PULL BACK

PREREQUISITES: Hamstring Stretch 2 (Exercise 9-2), Thigh Stretch 3: Kneeling (Exercise 13), Leg Pull Front (Exercise 54).

PURPOSE: To mobilize the hip joints, stretch the hamstrings, and stabilize the shoulders.

EXERCISE DESCRIPTION:

Starting Position: This position is the opposite of the push-up. With the chest facing the ceiling, extend the arms below the shoulders. Keep the shoulders, hips, and heels in a straight line, the toes pointed, the chin to the rib cage, the pelvis slightly tucked under (posteriorly), and the shoulder blades pressed to the hips.

a) Do the B-Line and flex your right foot. Breathe in as you kick one leg to the ceiling (and past the vertical line if you can), pulling the abdominals in tighter. Keep the hips pressed to the ceiling, lift the chest to the ceiling, and lengthen the back of the neck. Keep the shoulders relaxed, the ribs to the hips, and the abdominals firm.

b) Point the foot of the raised leg and breathe out as you slowly lower the leg to the floor.

c) Touch lightly on the floor and kick the same leg again.

ADVANCED: At the top of the kick, do a double kick and a double breath in.

KEY POINTS: Keep the pelvis lifted up as the leg kicks up. Elongate the head and neck out of the shoulders. Be sure that the pressure on the supporting leg is in the center of the heel.

CARE: Imagine there is a rod from the center top of your shoulders to the tailbone and another across your shoulders. Avoid hyperextending the elbows.

REPETITIONS: Five kicks on one leg, then five kicks on the other.

BREATHING: Breathe in on the kick up, and breathe out on the return.

NOTES

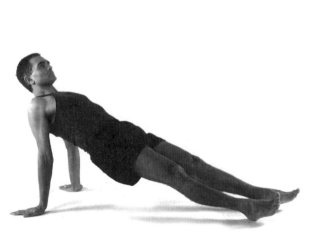
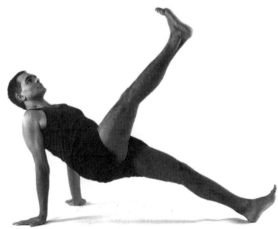

Exercise 56
SIDE KICK 2

PREREQUISITES: The Start Stretches (Exercises 3 to 6a), The Hundreds: Alternating Legs (Exercise 31), Side Kick 1 (Exercise 49).

PURPOSE: To mobilize the hips, stretch the thighs, and strengthen the lower back.

EXERCISE DESCRIPTION:

Starting Position: Lie on the floor on your right side, and place your head in your right hand.

a) Keeping your legs straight, bring them slightly forward, with the top leg parallel and both feet flexed, and the bottom leg turned out with the toes pressed into the floor. Lengthen through the heels. Lift the left leg slightly to hip level, keep the foot flexed, and do the B-Line.

b) Take a deep breath in as you kick the leg forward as far as you can, pressing through the heel. Keep the spine straight. At the end of the kick, do an additional, smaller kick, inhaling an extra breath to expand the lungs further.

c) Point your foot and breathe out as you kick your leg back in a sweeping motion. As the top leg sweeps behind the straight line of the body, raise the torso up onto the right elbow, creating a large gap under your right armpit.

d) Flex the foot and press through the heel for the next kick forward. As the leg kicks forward again, lean back slightly to reduce the gap under the armpit, keeping the back as straight as possible, and flatten the rib cage.

ADVANCED: For the starting position, place your left hand behind your head, with the elbow to the ceiling in line with the body.

KEY POINTS: Stabilize your center and, as if your hip were the center of a circle, lengthen through the heel and toe, reaching past the outer rim of the circle. Keep the shoulders stable and the chin lifted. Lengthen through the crown of the head. To keep the top hip directly above the bottom one, create a small gap between the waist and the floor.

CARE: If you feel any strain in the back, discontinue the exercise. If you feel the hipbone on the mat, place a flat cushion under the hip.

REPETITIONS: Ten kicks on each side.

BREATHING: Breathe in as you kick forward, taking an extra breath in at the stretch. Breathe out as you kick back.

NOTES

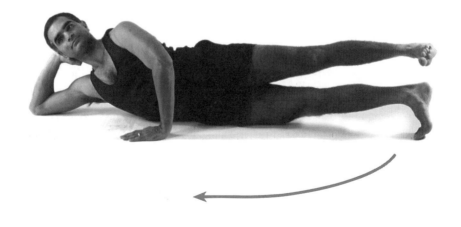

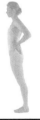

Exercise 57
BOOMERANG

PREREQUISITES: Teaser 2 (Exercise 53-2), The Roll-Over (or Spine Roll) (Exercise 34).

PURPOSE: To gain control and mobilization of the spine, shoulders, and hips, and to stretch the hamstrings.

EXERCISE DESCRIPTION:

Starting Position: Do the B-Line and sit upright on the floor, imagining that you have a rod through your spine. Place your palms on the floor by the hips, and extend your legs forward, locked at the knee joint, with the right ankle crossed over the left.

a) Tuck the pelvis slightly, take a deep breath out as you sink into your hips, and roll back, drawing the thighs to the ribs into a roll-over until the feet almost touch the mat. Lengthen the neck and roll only to the top of the shoulders (Figure i).

b) Squeezing the inner thighs, quickly cross the legs the other way (left over right).

c) Breathe in as you roll forward, extending your arms off the floor, out to the sides, and behind your back. Try to hold the left hand with the right, keeping the elbows locked, and continue to extend the hands behind you and up toward the ceiling.

d) Balance on your sit bones for three seconds with the legs 12 inches off the floor, spine erect, legs straight (Figure ii).

e) Breathe out as you continue the roll forward, lengthening your chest toward your knees and your head toward your feet, with your hands extended and pressing to the ceiling (Figure iii).

f) Breathe in as you release the hands and stretch them around in a circle to the ceiling, rotating the shoulder joints. At the same time curl the torso into the upright sitting position, placing the hands by the hips.

KEY POINTS: The entire movement centers around contracted and controlled abdominal strength, precision, and flowing movement.

CARE: Roll back only onto the tops of the shoulders. Keep the shoulder blades pressed to the hips and the neck straight and long when clasping the hands behind the back.

REPETITIONS: One set of up to eight complete movements.

BREATHING: Breathe in as you sit tall, and breathe out as you roll over. Breathe in as you roll up to balance. Hold for three seconds. Breathe out as you roll and reach the chest to the knees. Breathe in as you extend to the upright position.

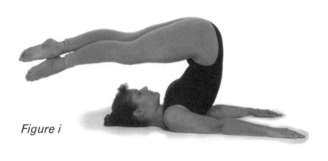

Figure i

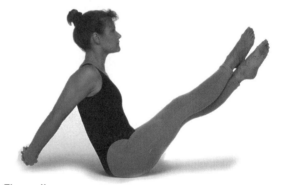

Figure ii

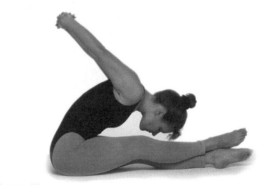

Figure iii

Exercise 58
SEAL

PREREQUISITE: The Roll-Over (or Spine Roll) (Exercise 34).

PURPOSE: To gain balance and control of movement and to stretch the spine.

EXERCISE DESCRIPTION:

Starting Position: Sit tall on the mat, with the knees bent and open, the elbows placed on the inside of the thighs, the forearms under the calves and holding onto the front of the ankles, and the arms straight. Place the soles of the feet together, and raise the heels off the mat, but keep the toes lightly touching the mat.

a) Do the B-Line and breathe out as you tuck the pelvis to start to roll the spine. Continue to smoothly roll over onto the top of the shoulders until the heels are 2 inches off the mat.

b) Balancing in this position, open the feet 8 inches and clap them together three times.

c) Breathe in as you roll into the starting position, straightening the spine at the top of the roll, toes just off the mat, and clap the soles of the feet three times.

KEY POINTS: Keep the neck long, and keep the ribs to the hips on the roll back. When balancing on the shoulders, keep the abdominals hollow and firm.

CARE: Keep the shoulder blades pressed to the hips to avoid neck strain.

REPETITIONS: One set of up to eight repetitions.

BREATHING: Breathe in as you sit in a continuous C curve. Breathe out as you roll back. Hold your breath for the three claps. Breathe in as you roll up.

NOTES

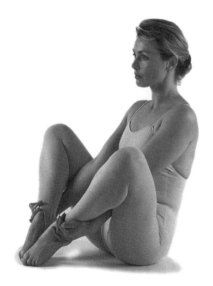

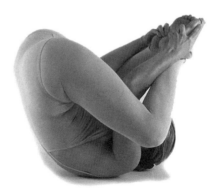

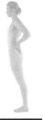

Exercise 59
CONTROL BALANCE

PREREQUISITE: The Roll-Over (or Spine Roll) (Exercise 34).

PURPOSE: To gain control, balance, coordination, and abdominal strength.

EXERCISE DESCRIPTION:

Starting Position: Lie on your back with your arms above your head on the floor, legs vertical and parallel.

a) Do the B-Line and breathe out as you roll over until the toes touch the mat, with the tailbone to the ceiling. Hold on to the right ankle with both hands.

b) Breathe in as you extend the left leg to the ceiling, past the vertical line of the hip, extending through the toes. Keep the leg turned out and the foot pointed. Extend the spine as upright as possible, pressing the tailbone to the ceiling and the toes of the right foot into the floor above your head.

c) Breathe in as you release the right ankle, and smoothly scissor the legs, keeping the torso and legs under control. Keep the tailbone lengthened to the ceiling.

d) Breathe out as you extend the right leg to the ceiling, turned out and pointed. Holding onto the left ankle, with the leg straight, press the toes into the mat and lengthen through the heel.

KEY POINTS: By pressing the heel to the mat, you can achieve a better stretch up the back of the leg. Keep the extended leg to the ceiling, locked at the knee joint. Consciously think of releasing the front of the thigh.

CARE: Keep the shoulders open and on the mat, and the neck lengthened. This will provide more stability for the movement. Keep the abdominals hollow and the back straight.

REPETITIONS: One set of six extensions on each leg.

BREATHING: Breathe out as the leg extends to the ceiling. Breathe in as the legs change direction.

NOTES

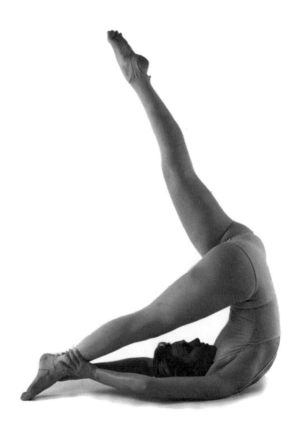

CHAPTER 9

The Advanced Routine

As small bricks are employed

to build large buildings, so will

the development of small muscles

help develop large muscles.

J. PILATES

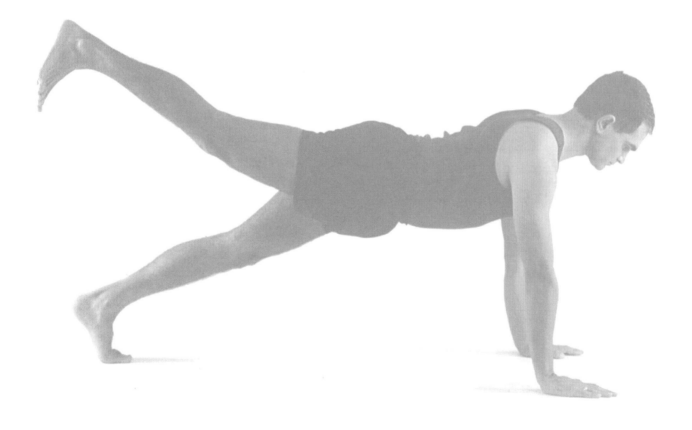

PREREQUISITE: The Hundreds: Alternating Legs (Exercise 31).

PURPOSE: To strengthen the abdominals with increased body extension.

EXERCISE DESCRIPTION: Start in the same position as for the Hundreds (Exercise 31). Keep the feet pointed and turned out.

a) Do the B-Line and breathe out as you lower the legs down to eye level (or as close to that as you can get comfortably) for a five-second count, at the same time still trying to lift your buttocks off the floor for stronger, lower abdominal connection.

b) Point the feet, do the B-Line harder, and breathe in as you raise the legs back to the vertical position, squeezing the inner thighs.

KEY POINTS: Same as those for the previous Hundreds, as well as the following: When lowering the legs, squeeze the inner thighs and allow the abdominal muscles to slowly release; this will allow the legs to lower without the back arching. Then anchor the abdominals before lifting the legs, and imagine the hips drawing to the ribs; the contraction of the abdominals is what brings the legs back to the vertical position. Squeeze the inner thighs. As you lower the legs, be sure not to lower the head and shoulders, as this will arch the back (it might help to look in a mirror to check the stability of the torso).

CARE: If, after lowering or raising the legs, you feel as if the abdominals have had enough, return to the resting position.

REPETITIONS: Two sets of ten, with a five-second rest between each set.

NOTES

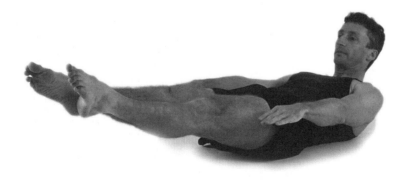

Exercise 61
ROLL-OVER: BENT LEGS

PREREQUISITES: The Roll-Over (or Spine Roll) (Exercise 34), Rolling (Exercise 37).

PURPOSE: To connect the deeper abdominal muscles, especially in the lower abdominal section.

EXERCISE DESCRIPTION:

Starting Position: Lie on the floor with your back flat, the knees bent to the chest and shoulder-distance apart, and the ankles crossed.

a) Do the B-Line and, attempting to keep your heels as close as you can to your buttocks, breathe out as you roll the hips off the floor to your ribs. Draw your knees close to your chest and in toward your armpits.

b) Roll onto the shoulders only, lengthening your neck.

c) Breathe into your upper back as you hold the position.

d) Breathe out as you slowly roll back, imprinting your spine onto the floor, and slowly release the abdominals to prevent the head and shoulders lifting off the floor.

KEY POINTS: If you are unable to perform the exercise with the heels to the tailbone, lengthen the legs until you gain more control. It is on the roll down that you will feel the lower abdominals connecting. Continue the repetitions without any rest. Keep the thighs close to the body at all times.

CARE: Roll onto the shoulders only, not the neck. Start this exercise with your legs long and bent, ankles crossed. As you become more proficient, keep the heels closer to the tailbone. The last 25 percent of the exercise, on the release, is the most challenging part to control.

REPETITIONS: One set of ten, with the ankles crossed each way after each roll.

NOTES

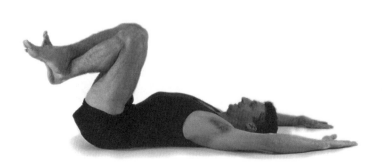

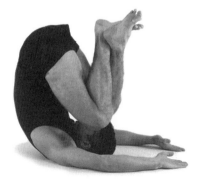

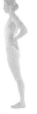

Exercise 62
PENDULUM

PREREQUISITE: Corkscrew 2: Advanced (Exercise 47-2).

PURPOSE: To strengthen the obliques and abdominals, and to mobilize and strengthen the spine.

EXERCISE DESCRIPTION:

Starting Position: Lie on your back on the floor, with the legs straight to the ceiling, turned out, and the feet pointed. Keep the arms above the head, elbows bent and pressed into the mat, and hands slightly more than shoulder-distance apart. (In the basic version, the hands are by the sides, as shown in the figure.)

a) Do the B-Line and, keeping the feet together, breathe out as you move your legs over to the right in line with your navel. Lift the left hip off the floor. Keep the shoulder blades and elbows pressed into the mat.

b) Draw the hips to the ribs and breathe in as you roll the back of the left side of the rib cage back onto the floor. Then continue with the rest of the spine until the left hip presses into the floor.

c) Keep moving to the other side without stopping. Turn the head in the opposite direction from the legs.

KEY POINTS: Keep the legs turned out, especially when returning to the vertical position. Release the opposite chest muscle to allow the shoulder to stay on the mat.

CARE: If there is too much pressure on the arms to raise the legs back to the vertical position, then the legs have gone over too far. When over to the side, draw the legs up to the elbow to keep the abdominals connected and prevent the back from arching. Keep the toes in line with the navel.

As you develop more control, take the legs farther over to the sides to a distance of several inches off the floor without lifting the shoulder blades at all. Well done if you are able to do this without straining!

REPETITIONS: One set of ten on each side, alternating sides.

NOTES

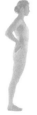

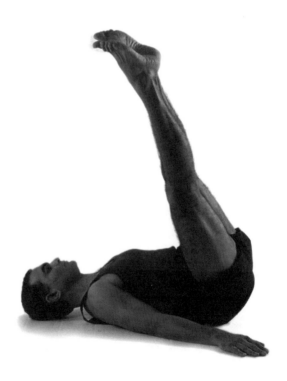

The Advanced Routine

PREREQUISITES: The Hundreds: Lower and Raise (Exercise 60), The Perfect Abdominal Curl (Exercise 25) with straight legs.

PURPOSE: To improve abdominal control and strength.

EXERCISE DESCRIPTION:

Starting Position: Lie on your back on the floor, legs extended 15 inches apart in front of you, feet flexed, knees pressed into the floor. Place your hands behind your head, with the fingers interlocked, and your elbows on the mat (Figure i).

a) Do the B-Line and breathe in as you raise the head and shoulders off the mat, keeping the elbows behind the ears, as if a bar were passing in front of the elbows and behind the head (Figure ii).

b) Breathe out as you curl forward, contracting the ribs to the hips, "zipping up" the stomach. Reach forward as far as you can, trying to extend your chest to your knees.

c) Breathe in as you imprint your spine up an imaginary wall into the upright position. Lift the ribs out of the hips without hunching the shoulders (Figure iii).

d) Breathe out as you sink into the hips, tucking the pelvis to connect the lower abdominals, press through the heels, and imprint your spine on the mat, keeping the ribs to the hips until the shoulder blades rest on the mat (Figure ii).

e) Extend the neck onto the mat, maintaining the B-Line.

KEY POINTS: Zip up the stomach before you start to lift the head. Keep the elbows open. Keep the shoulder blades pressed to the hips. Peel your spine off the mat.

CARE: Breathe out 75 percent of your capacity in the first 25 percent of the movements up or down. Flatten the ribs to the floor before rolling the shoulders off the mat. Keep the chin slightly off the chest. Do not pull on the neck, and always keep the elbows wide open.

REPETITIONS: One set of up to ten.

BREATHING: Breathe in as the head and shoulders lift upright. Breathe out as you roll up and forward. Breathe in as you imprint to the vertical position. Breathe out as you roll down.

NOTES

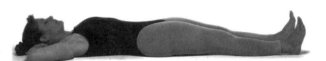

Figure i

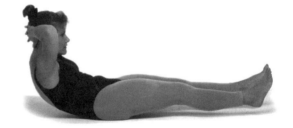

Figure ii

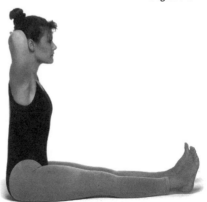

Figure iii

Exercise 64
JACKKNIFE

PREREQUISITES: Roll-Over: Bent Legs (Exercise 61), Helicopter Hundreds (Exercise 70), The Perfect Abdominal Curl (Exercise 25) with straight legs.

PURPOSE: To stretch the spine, stretch the neck, and increase abdominal control.

EXERCISE DESCRIPTION:

Starting Position: Lie on your back, palms down, legs extended vertically, toes pointed and parallel (Figure i).

a) Breathe out as you roll over onto the shoulders without allowing the legs to lower to the floor (Figure ii).

b) Immediately lengthen the legs to a vertical position as if the body were in a straight line to the ceiling. Extend through the toes, squeeze the inner thighs, and hold the buttocks firmly. Press your hips toward a straight line above your eyes (Figure iii).

c) Balance and hold the position for the breath in.

d) Breathe out as you slowly imprint your spine on the mat, trying to keep your feet above your eyes until the hips have lengthened away from the ribs and pressed into the mat (Figure iv).

e) Breathe in as you lower the legs toward the floor to a level where the back remains flat (in the B-Line).

f) Repeat.

KEY POINTS: Keep the shoulders relaxed, without putting much pressure into the hands. The jackknife over is a fast movement, but you should come slowly down from it. Maintain total focus on flat, strong abdominals at all times.

CARE: Keep the neck as long as possible. Avoid this exercise unless you feel 100 percent confident

that you can completely control the movement. The movement must be smooth and elegant throughout.

REPETITIONS: One set of up to eight repetitions.

BREATHING: Breathe out as you jackknife over and up to the vertical position. Balance and breathe into the upper back. Breathe out on the roll down.

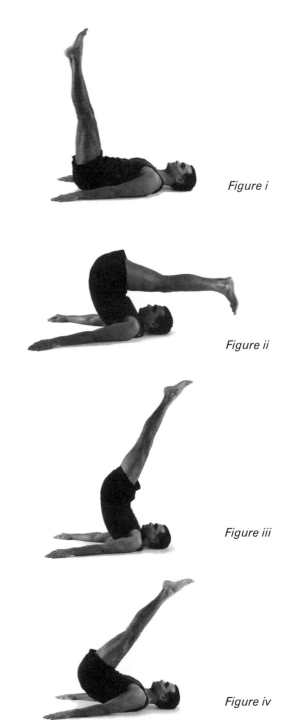

Figure i

Figure ii

Figure iii

Figure iv

PREREQUISITES: The Hundreds: Alternating Legs (Exercise 31), Roll-Over: Bent Legs (Exercise 61), Jackknife (Exercise 64).

PURPOSE: To increase abdominal control, stretch the upper back and neck, mobilize the hips, and stretch the hip flexors.

EXERCISE DESCRIPTION:

Starting Position: Lie on your back with your legs extended, hands by your sides, palms down.

a) Do the B-Line and breathe out as you do a jackknife (Exercise 64) to the ceiling. In the vertical position, place your hands into the small of your back to support your hips in an upright position; keep the elbows pressed on the mat and close to each other.

b) Keeping the knees locked, toes pointed, and buttocks held firmly, breathe out as you stretch the right leg away from your head past the point of the elbows toward the floor. At the same time, lower and stretch the left leg past your head so that the left knee is in line with your eyes (see Figure).

c) Breathe in as you bring both legs to the vertical position, squeezing the inner thighs, and smoothly change over.

d) Breathe out as you change legs.

KEY POINTS: As the leg stretches past the point of the elbows (and the vertical line to the ceiling), draw the hipbones to the rib cage. You will feel the abdominals connect more, which will minimize any tendency to arch the back. A triangle of your hands, elbows, and shoulders provides the infrastructure for the position of the movement. The control is always firmly from the center with the ribs flat.

CARE: Keep the neck relaxed and lengthened. The hand should be lightly supporting the lower back, not providing the main support. The chin should be slightly off the chest so the breathing can flow easily.

REPETITIONS: One set of five on each side.

BREATHING: Breathe out on the scissors. Breathe in on the close of the legs.

ADVANCED VERSION: Perform the scissors more rapidly. Breathe in for two scissors and breathe out for two scissors: in, in (stretch, stretch) out, out (stretch, stretch).

NOTES

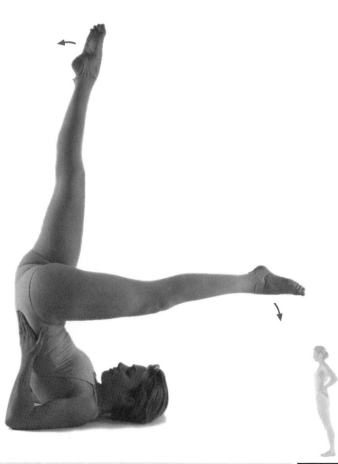

Exercise 66
BICYCLE

PREREQUISITE: Scissors (Exercise 65).

PURPOSE: To mobilize the hip joints, keep the abdominals long and strong, stretch the hip flexors, and stabilize the pelvic area.

EXERCISE DESCRIPTION:

Starting Position: The starting position is the same as for the Scissors. Once you have attained the upright position, go on to the following steps:

    a) B-Line and breathe out as you extend the left leg past the point of the elbows and bend the knee to reach the toes toward the floor (see Figure).

    b) Breathe in with the left knee drawn toward eye level and extended to the ceiling. Extend the right leg past the point of the elbows and down to the floor, while the left foot extends to the ceiling with the knee above the eyes.

The action is like that of pedaling a bicycle (hence, the name of the exercise).

KEY POINTS: Consciously stretch the front of the thigh as you extend the leg and bend the knee, pointing the toe to the floor. Imagine the area from the hip to the rib being stretched. As the knee draws toward eye level, keep the abdominals firm. Do not draw the knee toward the face or chest; keep the cycling action away from the chest.

CARE: As the foot extends to the floor, keep any excessive pressure off the hands in order to avoid placing more pressure on the lower back.

REPETITIONS: One set of five cycling motions with each leg.

BREATHING: Breathe out as the leg stretches to the floor. Breathe in for the cycle movement.

NOTES

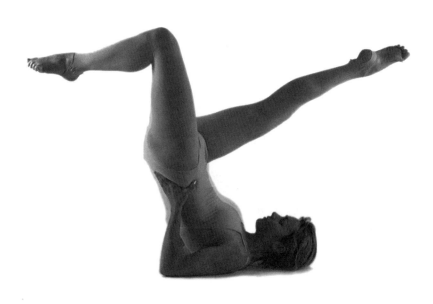

Exercise 67
SHOULDER BRIDGE

PREREQUISITE: The Hundreds: Alternating Legs (Exercise 31).

PURPOSE: To extend the lower back while providing support for the abdominals, and to stretch the hip flexors.

EXERCISE DESCRIPTION:

Starting Position: Lie on your back with the knees bent, feet parallel, hands by your sides.

a) B-Line and breathe out as you curl the hips up from the mat, lengthen the neck, and support the back by placing one hand under each hip, elbows under the hands, feet firmly pressed into the mat.

b) Breathe out as you point the right foot and stretch it as close to the floor as you can until the leg is straight, with the knee locked.

c) Breathe in as you quickly kick through the stretched right toe as high and as far back above the head as you can. Flex the foot toward the end of the kick, keeping the hips immobile.

d) Breathe out as you slowly lower the right leg to the floor with the flexed foot. Press the heel as far as you can to the ground, then point the foot and repeat.

KEY POINTS: Keep the buttocks gently held together. The shoulders, elbows, and feet support the position. Hold the abdominals firmly, with the ribs to the hips. When lowering the leg, stretch the top of the thigh, "zip up" the stomach, and imagine you are tucking the pelvis under to open the lower back.

CARE: Keep the lower back as open as possible, especially when the leg lowers to the floor. Do the B-Line firmly.

REPETITIONS: Five kicks with the right leg, five kicks with the left.

BREATHING: Breathe out as you stretch to the floor. Breathe in as you kick. Breathe out as you lower and stretch the leg.

NOTES

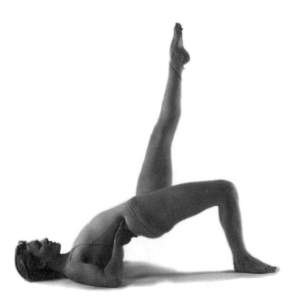

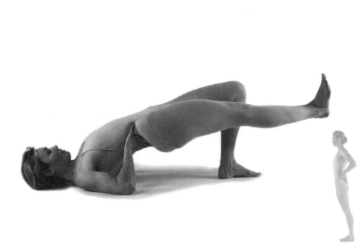

Exercise 68
CAN-CAN

PREREQUISITES: The Hundreds: Alternating Legs (Exercise 31), Side to Side (Exercise 23).

PURPOSE: To mobilize the lower back and hips.

EXERCISE DESCRIPTION:

Starting Position: Sit upright with your hands behind you on the floor, elbows straight. Place your feet close to your buttocks, with the toes pointed and touching the floor. Keep the knees together.

a) Do the B-Line and, breathing out, let both knees lower to the floor to the left. The right buttock may rise off the floor.

b) Do the B-Line harder and, breathing in, raise both knees back to the starting position by drawing the front of the right hip to the floor.

c) Repeat to the other side, gradually getting the knees closer to the floor each time.

KEY POINTS: Keep the shoulders and upper torso as still as possible. On each movement to the side, feel the lower back on that side opening. Squeeze the inner thighs.

CARE: If you feel any twinge or strain in the lower back, do not lower the knees too far to the side.

REPETITIONS: Ten repetitions on each side.

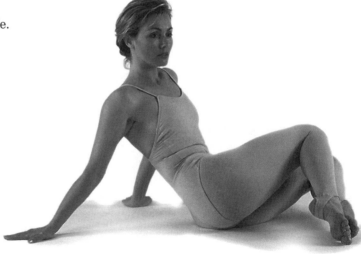

Exercise 68-1
CAN-CAN EXTENSION

PREREQUISITE: Can-Can (Exercise 68).

PURPOSE: To mobilize and strengthen the lower back, hips, and lower abdominals.

EXERCISE DESCRIPTION: This is the advanced version of the Can-Can, with some additions.

Starting Position: As in the Can-Can.

  a) After lowering the knees to the side (less than your normal distance), do the B-Line and breathe in as you then extend the legs (still keeping them together) into the air.

  b) Breathe out as you draw the heels back to your tailbone and continue as in the Can-Can to the other side.

KEY POINTS: Try not to lean back as the legs extend. Keep the arms and back as straight as possible.

CARE: At first, the thighs may feel as if they are gripping on the extension, but this will gradually ease. Stop at a comfortable number of repetitions if you are unable to complete ten.

REPETITIONS: Ten on each side.

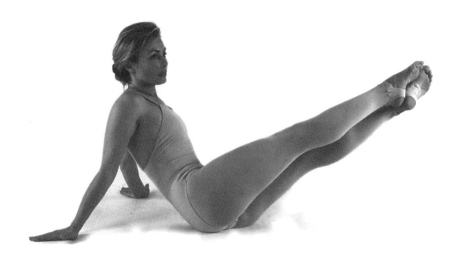

Exercise 69
HIP CIRCLES

This is similar to the advanced Corkscrew, but it is done in a seated position.

PREREQUISITES: Corkscrew 2: Advanced (Exercise 47-2), Pendulum (Exercise 62), Can-Can Extension (Exercise 68-1).

PURPOSE: To increase abdominal and hip flexor strength, hip joint mobility, and lower back mobility.

EXERCISE DESCRIPTION:

Starting Position: Sit upright on the mat. Keeping your spine as straight as possible, lean back with your hands behind you in a 45 degree angle. Keep the hands wide apart and the elbows locked.

a) Do the B-Line, bend your knees to the chest, and extend them to the ceiling, with the feet pointed. Squeeze the inner thighs.

b) Breathe out as you swing the legs around in a circle to the right, down to just off the mat, and then around to the left.

c) Breathe in as you squeeze the inner thighs and stretch the toes to the ceiling, trying to keep the thighs as close to your chest as possible.

d) Repeat in the other direction.

KEY POINTS: Lengthen the neck out of the shoulders, as if someone were lengthening you up from the crown of your head. Keep the chest open and maintain the B-Line at all times. "Zip up" the stomach as you raise the legs up to the ceiling. Keep the hips as square as you can. The hips will slightly rise off the floor as you go to the sides. As the legs lower to the floor, flatten the ribs to the hips, keeping the spine long. Lengthen through the toes.

CARE: If you feel strain in the wrists or shoulders, discontinue the exercise. Do not hunch the shoulders.

REPETITIONS: Up to five Hip Circles in each direction.

BREATHING: Breathe out on the lower part of the circle. Breathe in as you raise the legs to the ceiling.

NOTES

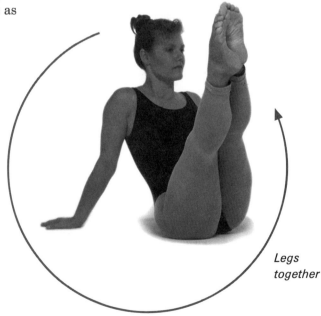

Legs together

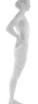

Exercise 70
HELICOPTER HUNDREDS

PREREQUISITE: The Hundreds: Alternating Legs (Exercise 31).

PURPOSE: To strengthen the abdominals and mobilize the hip joints.

EXERCISE DESCRIPTION:

Starting Position: Lie on your back on the floor, with the knees to the chest and the hands on the ankles.

a) Do the B-Line and breathe out as you contract forward, arms extended just off the floor past the hips; keep the legs vertical, with the feet pointed and turned out.

b) Scissor (or split) the legs, with the left leg to the ceiling and the right leg to the floor. Then breathe in as you take the legs around in a circle in opposite directions, away from the body, keeping the legs turned out and the feet pointed. The right leg opens to the side and comes up to the vertical position; the left leg opens to the side and lowers to just off the floor.

c) Breathe out as you scissor the legs.

d) Repeat five times in each direction.

KEY POINTS: Lengthen out of the hip sockets as much as possible, maintaining your turnout. Focus on the inner thigh (adductor) muscles to make the circle.

CARE: If the hips joints "click," either lengthen out of the hip joints further, reduce the range of movement of the circle, or reduce the turnout of the leg.

REPETITIONS: Repeat five times, then change direction.

BREATHING: Breathe out as you lower and "split" the legs. Breathe in as you circle the legs.

NOTES

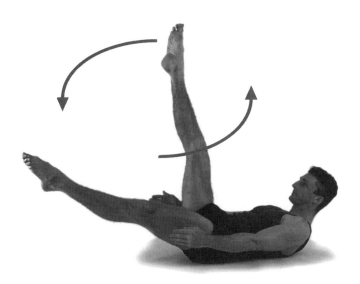
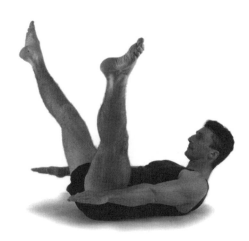
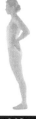

Exercise 71
LYING TORSO STRETCH

PREREQUISITE: Side to Side (Exercise 23).

PURPOSE: This is a cooling-down stretch. It mobilizes the middle and upper back and shoulders and releases tension in the lower back.

EXERCISE DESCRIPTION:

Starting Position: Lying on your right side, straighten the right leg and bend the left leg so it is lying on the floor in front of you, with the left heel touching the right knee. Lengthen the right arm in front of the chest, with the palm up. Stretch the left arm out in front of the chest, reaching as far as possible through the fingertips, past the right hand; lean the left shoulder forward.

a) Do the B-Line and breathe in as you scrape the floor with the fingers of the left hand, making a circle until the arm is above the head.

b) Breathe out as you then complete the circle, taking the left arm behind the body, palm upward, turning the head to the ceiling. Turn the left shoulder backward to face the ceiling and open the left armpit to the ceiling. Keep the left knee on the ground.

c) Begin to complete the circle by taking the left hand toward the right foot and forward in front of the chest to the starting position.

KEY POINTS: As the shoulder loosens and the upper back becomes more flexible, the circling hand may eventually touch the floor for the movement. As the arm extends behind the body, lengthen the entire body from the toes of the lower leg through the fingertips of the circling arm. If the muscles feel tight during a particular point of the stretch, stay in that position for several seconds to release the tension before continuing.

CARE: Do not try to force the top shoulder down to the floor. Allow the body to release into the stretch gradually.

REPETITIONS: One set of ten repetitions of five circles in each direction.

NOTES

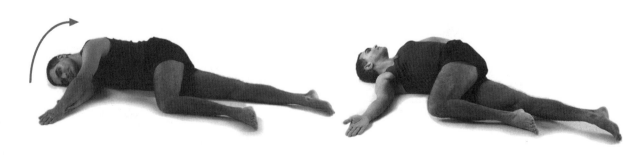

Exercise 72
STANDING SIDE STRETCHES: BASIC

PREREQUISITE: None.

PURPOSE: To stretch the muscles down the side of the body from the armpit to the hip.

EXERCISE DESCRIPTION:

Starting Position: Stand to the side of the frame of a doorway about 12 inches away from the edge of the frame so it is on your right-hand side. Hold on to the door frame with the right hand just below hip level. Take the left hand over the head and hold onto the frame at approximately forehead level.

a) B-Line: Breathe out and stretch the body away from the frame as far as possible. Straighten the top arm. Press the left hip to the floor and the left lower ribs to the ceiling. Turn the armpit toward the ceiling for a much greater stretch of the muscle near the shoulder blade (latissimus dorsi).

b) Breathe in without moving, then breathe out and stretch a little farther.

c) After five stretches, do the B-Line harder and use the abdominals to return to the upright position. Do not use the arms. Change sides and repeat the movement.

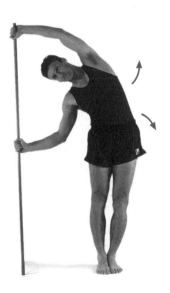

d) To achieve a greater stretch and increase the effectiveness of the stretch, press the right hand against the frame, without hunching the right shoulder.

KEY POINTS: Relax the inside shoulder. Allow the head to relax under the right arm, and look straight ahead.

CARE: After stretching to the side, turn the hips slightly in (with the outside hip slightly in front of the inside hip) to avoid any pressure on the back. It the lower back feels tight during the exercise, tuck the pelvis under to open up the lower back. You might also feel a stretch just above the hip in the lower back area.

REPETITIONS: Two sets of ten breaths in and out per side, alternating after each five. Use the B-Line and not the arms when returning to the upright position after the ten breaths.

Exercise 72-1
STANDING SIDE STRETCHES: ADVANCED

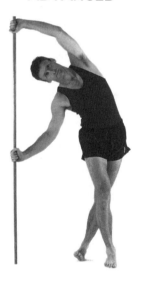

Add the following after the final step in Exercise 72: Place the left leg behind the right leg on the outside edge of the left heel. Bend the right leg and continue as above. This will give a greater stretch to the top outside of the hip.

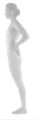

Exercise 73
CAT STRETCH

PREREQUISITE: None.

PURPOSE: To increase flexion mobility of the spine.

EXERCISE DESCRIPTION:

Starting Position: Kneel on all fours, with the knees and hands shoulder-distance apart. Relax the head in line with the spine.

    a) Breathe out as you slowly draw the head to the groin while pressing the spine to the ceiling.

    b) Breathe in as you release the ribs away from the hips until the spine is horizontal to the floor. Lengthen the hips away from the ribs.

KEY POINTS: Attempt to draw your nose to your B-Line and your hips to your ribs in the same movement. This will stretch the cervical, thoracic, and lumbar areas of the spine.

CARE: If there is too much mobility in the upper back, concentrate more on drawing the hips to the ribs. This exercise is great for pregnant women (see figures), as it stretches the tight lower back muscles.

REPETITIONS: Ten stretches.

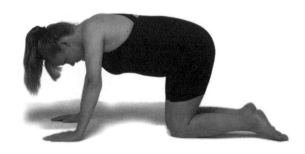
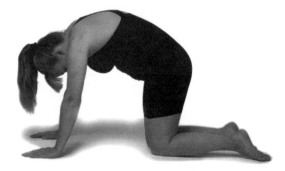

Exercise 74
ROCKING

PREREQUISITES: Thigh Stretches (Exercises 11 to 13), Swan Dive 2 (Exercise 42-1). A strong back is required!

PURPOSE: To control and stretch the front (anterior) part of the body, and to work and strengthen the back muscles.

EXERCISE DESCRIPTION:

Starting Position: Lie prone on the mat and draw your heels to your buttocks, and move the knees shoulder-width apart, with the feet slightly closer. Reach behind you and hold the outsides of the feet with your hands. Keep the shoulder blades pressed to the hips and extend the crown of the head toward the line of the toes.

  a) Do the B-Line and, as you breathe out, roll forward onto the chest, keeping your chin off the floor.

  b) Breathe in as you rock backward as hard as you can, opening the chest and lifting it off the mat. Keep the buttocks tight.

  c) Breathe out and repeat the exercise.

KEY POINTS: Think of your spine like the curved legs of a rocking chair. Rock and elongate through the tips of the knees and the top of the chest. Keep the spine as long and open as possible. Flatten the rib cage on the roll forward so it does not poke into the mat. Keep the abdominals hollow and firm.

CARE: If the back feels any pressure, stop the exercise. Keep the shoulders open and down to the hips.

REPETITIONS: One set of up to eight rocking movements.

BREATHING: Breathe out as you roll forward. Breathe in as you roll onto the thighs.

NOTES

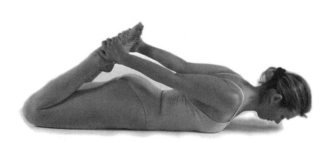
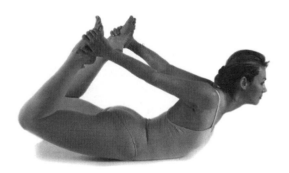

Exercise 75-1
TWIST 1

PREREQUISITES: Hamstring Stretch 3 (Exercise 10), Pendulum (Exercise 62).

PURPOSE: To increase rotation of the spine, open the lower back, and mobilize and strengthen the shoulder girdle.

EXERCISE DESCRIPTION:

Starting Position: Sit partially on your right hip, knees toward the chest, left ankle over the right. Place the sole of the left foot flat on the mat, toes pointing forward, heels close to the tailbone. Place the right arm close to the right hip, with the palm pressed into the mat, pointed slightly forward. Lean slightly forward over the hand. Relax the left hand on the left ankle.

a) Do the B-Line and breathe in as you lift your tailbone to the ceiling as if you were being lifted by a piece of string attached to this point. The balance control is from the palm of the right hand and the sole of the left foot.

b) As the tailbone extends upward, reach through the fingertips of the left hand away from the body, in a smooth arc up to the ceiling and over toward the floor close to the left ear. The crown of the head and the fingers of the left hand should be reaching to the mat.

c) Breathe in as you reverse the movement, connecting the abdominals as if you were still being pulled by the tailbone to the ceiling. Extend the left arm as if you were drawing a line on the ceiling with your fingertips.

KEY POINTS: Reach the fingers of the moving arm, with the elbow joint unlocked, as if you were trying to touch the ceiling in both directions. Lift the tailbone as high as you can, trying to straighten the spine, keeping the abdominals hollow. Keep the shoulder blades in line with the hips. The movement is smooth and flowing, as if it were being performed by a ballet dancer.

CARE: To achieve balance in this exercise, you need to do the following: Place equal pressure on the heel and fingertips of the right hand. Keep a tripod on the left foot. The control emanates from the abdominals and from the stability of the right shoulder.

REPETITIONS: One set of five on each side.

BREATHING: Breathe in on the extension to the ceiling. Breathe out on the return to the mat.

NOTES

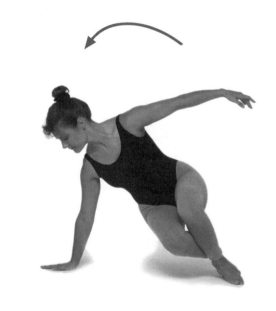

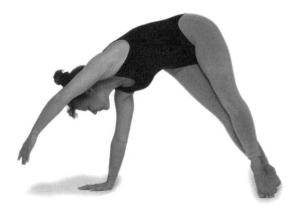

PREREQUISITE: Twist 1 (Exercise 75-1).

PURPOSE: To achieve advanced balance and control.

EXERCISE DESCRIPTION:

Starting Position: Sit upright on the mat, legs extended; place your right hand on the floor slightly behind you and lean over onto the right hip so that your torso faces away from the upright position. Cross the left leg on top of the right leg. Relax the left hand on the floor in front of the thigh (Figure i).

a) Do the B-Line and breathe in as you lift the left hipbone vertically as if it were attached to a string drawing upward. The control comes from pressing the left sole into the floor as much as possible. Squeeze the inner thighs.

b) As the movement begins, extend the left hand (elbow unlocked) toward the left foot, then draw a line to the ceiling and over toward a point above the left ear. Maintain absolute control (Figure ii).

c) Breathe in as you rotate only the torso to face the floor by rotating the left shoulder blade toward the right hand. Feel the obliques on both sides connect. Keep the left arm in line with the ear and the left shoulder blade to the left hip.

d) Breathe in as you rotate the torso back and continue as if you were opening your chest to the ceiling. The obliques and the abdominals are still strongly connected. Stretch the top of the thighs (Figure iii).

e) Breathe out as you return to the start, reversing the movements in steps b) and a).

KEY POINTS: When lifting the hip to the ceiling you should achieve a straight line, as if along a pole from the feet, tailbone, spine, and crown of the head. Keep the pelvis tucked under for better lower abdominal connection (this is not usually visually apparent; it is the internal connection that is more important).

CARE: Maintain careful, smooth control on the rotation of the torso. It is a precise movement that requires every fiber of the body to be active and all your concentration to be focused for the best result.

REPETITIONS: One set of up to five Twists on each side.

BREATHING: Breathe in on the lift. Breathe out as you rotate to the floor and in as you rotate to the ceiling. Breathe out as you return to the starting position.

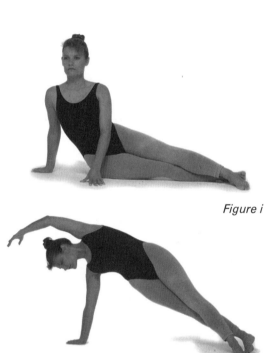

Figure i

Figure ii

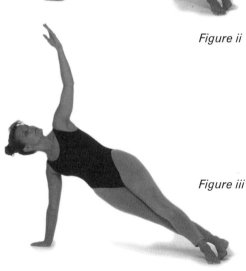

Figure iii

CHAPTER 10

More Advanced Exercises

When all your
muscles are properly
developed, you will,
as a matter of course,
perform your work with
minimum effort and
maximum pleasure.

J. PILATES

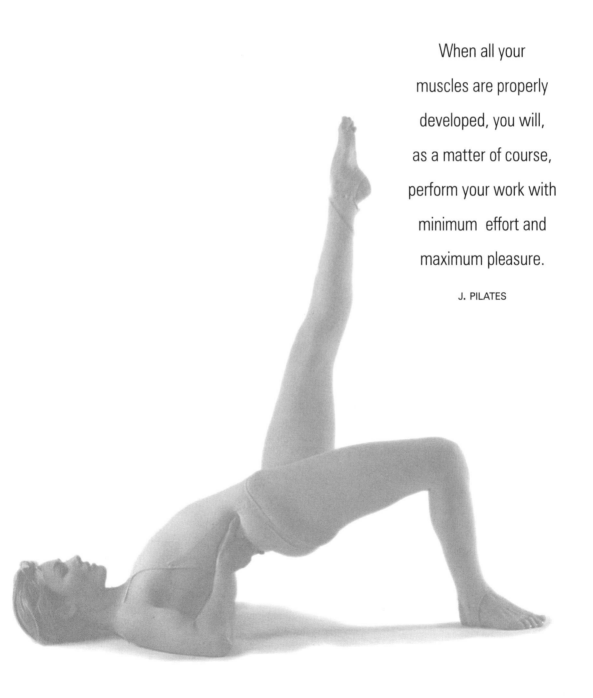

PREREQUISITE: The Perfect Abdominal Curl (Exercise 25).

PURPOSE: To strengthen the obliques. This is an advanced exercise.

EXERCISE DESCRIPTION: In essence, this exercise is the same as the Curl but with a twist.

Starting Position: Lie on the floor with the knees bent in a right angle at the knee joint, and contract forward with the hands behind the head and the elbows open.

a) Breathe out and draw the right shoulder toward the left knee, keeping the elbows open. Imagine you have a golf ball under your chin so you do not pull the head forward and strain the neck. Scoop the stomach.

b) Breathe in, release the torso until the shoulder blades almost touch the floor, and change sides.

c) Roll to the other side and repeat on that side.

KEY POINTS: Keep the shoulder blades off the floor at all times. Keep the elbows open. Turn the head and shoulders and look to the side for maximum rotation of the torso (where the eyes go, the body follows). Keep the hips still, planted into the mat. Maintain the B-Line at all times.

CARE: Keep the elbows open so there is less strain on the neck. Keep the chin off the chest, with the eyes forward at a 45-degree angle except when turning. When turning to the side, keep both shoulders off the floor.

REPETITIONS: One set of ten on each side.

Exercise 77
WRIST AND FOREARM STRENGTHENER

PREREQUISITE: None.

PURPOSE: To strengthen the wrists and forearms for all racquet sports and sports that require finger or wrist strength.

EXERCISE DESCRIPTION: Get a piece of thin rope approximately 5 feet long. Drill a hole through a wooden pole (12 inches long), pass the rope through the hole, and tie a knot at one end. Tie a weight of 4–8 lbs. or a bag of sand at the other end.

Starting Position: Stand up and, doing the B-Line, hold the pole at shoulder height in front of you, arms extended. If the weight is resting on the floor, make the rope shorter.

a) Always keeping the pole in the palm, slowly open the palm of the right hand and turn the wrist back to take hold of the underside of the pole. Grip the pole and rotate the right wrist forward as far as possible so that the knuckles are pointing toward the floor.

b) At the same time, turn the left wrist back and grip the pole. Now the left wrist extends forward as far as possible.

c) Keep repeating this procedure, taking the wrist through the extreme ranges of forward and backward motion until the rope has wound all the way up the pole. There should be enough pole for the rope to roll onto without hindering the hand grip. Breathe normally.

d) Once the rope is totally rolled up, reverse the wrist movement so you unroll the weight down to the floor. Do not let the pole slide through the fingers.

e) When the rope is unrolled, do not stop. Continue the unrolling action of the wrist so the rope once again begins to wind onto the pole. Repeat this movement up and down three times.

KEY POINTS: At the end of this exercise, the muscles in the forearm may feel as if they will burst through the skin because they are so pumped up! Rotate the wrists as fully forward and backward as possible. Do not let the ends of the pole swing up and down; keep it level to the floor throughout the exercise.

CARE: Vary the weight according to your requirements and strength. This is a challenge! Do as many wrist rolls of the rope as possible. At first, you may only be able to go up and down once. Aim for three times up and down. Adjust the weight if it becomes too easy. Keep the shoulders upright without hunching. Do not lean backward.

For those with weaker shoulders, this exercise can be done with the elbows by the sides and the forearms horizontal to the floor to start.

NOTES

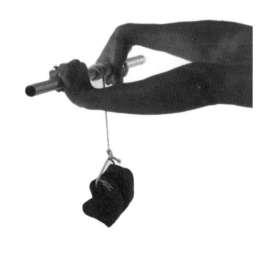

Exercise 78
NECK STRETCHES

PREREQUISITE: A tight neck!

PURPOSE: To loosen tight neck muscles.

EXERCISE DESCRIPTION:

Starting Position: Sit upright on a chair or on a bench (Figure i) on your sit bones. Place the feet hip-distance apart and planted on the floor. (Hold firmly onto the bench or onto one of the back legs of the chair, below seat level with the right hand.)

a) Breathe out and stretch the left ear to the left shoulder, pressing both shoulders to the floor. You should feel this stretch strongly on the right side of the neck.

b) Breathe out and, as the neck stretches to the side, slightly turn the head to the ceiling. You should feel this stretch slightly to the front of the neck.

KEY POINTS: The stretch should be mild at the beginning. Continue only if the feeling of the stretch is a good feeling.

CARE: If you feel any discomfort in the neck, stop the exercise.

REPETITIONS: Six to ten breaths in and out to each side of the head.

ADVANCED: You can obtain a stronger stretch by placing the opposite hand on the top of the head and slightly toward the ear of the side being stretched (Figure ii).

On the breath out, press the head against the pressure of the hand without the head moving. This isometric stretch will allow the neck muscles to lengthen further. Do not pull the head to the floor!

Breathe in and allow the head to relax further before repeating. Press the shoulder, on the side being stretched, firmly to the floor. The resistance from the hand on the head should be no more than 50 percent to start.

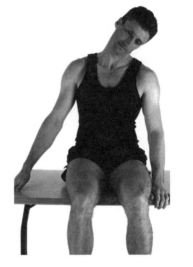

Figure i

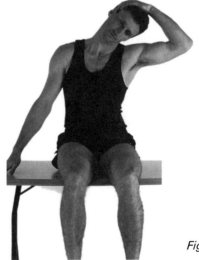

Figure ii

More Advanced Exercises

Exercise 79
SEATED SPINE ROTATION

PREREQUISITE: Side to Side (Exercise 23), Corkscrew 2: Advanced (Exercise 47-2) or Pendulum (Exercise 62).

PURPOSE: To stretch the tight muscles of the spine and obliques, and to increase rotational mobility.

EXERCISE DESCRIPTION:

Starting Position: Sit upright on a chair or on a bench (Figure i) on your sit bones. Place the feet hip-distance apart, planted on the floor. Place a long pole across the back of the shoulders parallel to the floor, and lengthen the arms along the pole with the hands holding on to the top of it.

a) Do the B-Line, breathe out, and stretch the left shoulder to a point behind you, keeping the arms horizontal and pressing both shoulders to the floor.

b) Breathe in as the torso returns to the central position.

c) Repeat to the other side.

KEY POINTS: The stretch should be mild at the beginning. Continue only if the feeling of the stretch is a good one. Turn the head around as much as you can: where the eyes go, the body follows! Keep the pole parallel to the floor at all times. Keep the shoulder blades pressed to the hips. Keep the hips square at all times.

CARE: If you feel any discomfort in the back, shoulders, or neck, stop the exercise.

REPETITIONS: Ten to each side. Once you are proficient with this exercise, you can speed up the movement.

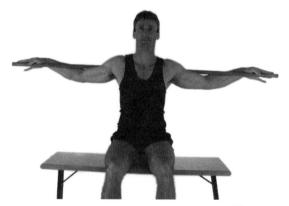

Figure i

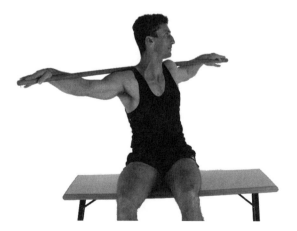

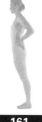

Figure ii

Exercise 80
CUSHION SQUEEZE

PREREQUISITE: None.

PURPOSE: To strengthen and tone the inner thighs (adductors).

EXERCISE DESCRIPTION:

Starting Position: Lie on your back on the floor with the knees bent and a firm cushion or several pillows placed between the knees. The feet should be flat on the floor about 12 inches apart.

a) Do the B-Line, and breathe out as you squeeze the cushion without tilting the pelvis or squeezing the buttocks.

b) Breathe in as you release only 10 percent of the squeeze before repeating.

KEY POINTS: The squeeze should be mild at the beginning. Gradually keep squeezing harder. To make the exercise even more effective, turn the toes in and feel the difference! This exercise can also be done with abdominal curls: curl up on the squeeze.

CARE: If there is any discomfort in the groin, stop. You should feel this exercise only in the inner thighs and not in the muscle attachments.

REPETITIONS: Two sets of ten squeezes, with a fifteen-second rest between each set.

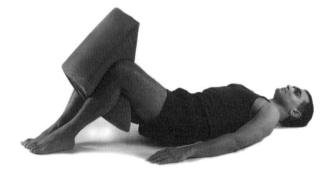

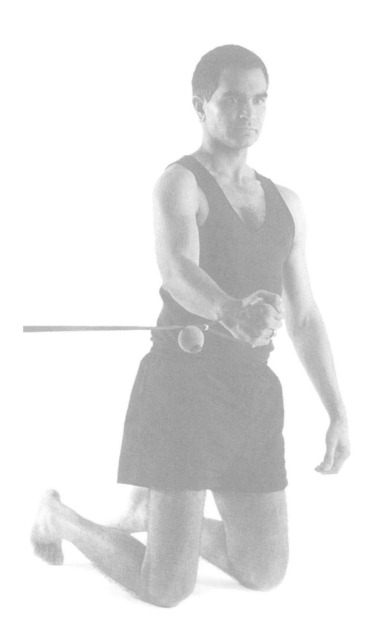

CHAPTER 11

Theraband Routines

Be certain that

you have your entire

body under complete

mental control.

J. PILATES

The following series of exercises is done with a length of Theraband or similar wide elastic. An Australian product called the IsoToner™ is particularly useful as it comes with a handle and cork balls for a better grip, as well as a piece of rope for locking into a door or tying to a door handle. (Please see the end of this book for information on purchasing the IsoToner™ product illustrated in these exercises.) There are no prerequisite exercises for this series, and anyone should be able to manage the exercises comfortably. As the Theraband comes in various strengths, there is a suitable resistance for everyone.

The photographs are straightforward and clearly illustrate the movements required. All of these exercises involve doing one to two sets of ten repetitions per side.

CAUTION: *Never pull the Theraband directly into your face.*

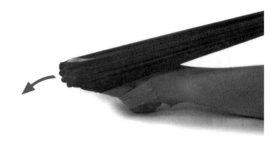

Exercise TB 2
POINTING THE TOES

This exercise strengthens the smaller muscles and tendons in the bottom of the foot, which are important for strengthening the toes. After the foot has extended through the ball of the foot, work only on flexion and extension of the toes, without flexing the foot at the ankle. Do not crunch the toes when extending. For ballet dancers, this is necessary for pointe work, jumping, and developing a pleasing line of the foot.

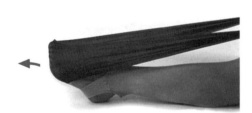

Exercise TB 1
POINTING THE FOOT
(PLANTAR FLEXION)

This exercise strengthens the calf muscles, the intrinsic muscles of the foot, and the ankle joint. Make sure that the toe is pointed in line with the knee. Using the muscles of the feet, press through the ball of the toe, stretching the top of the foot. These muscles are necessary for jumping, rising onto the ball of the foot, and balancing on the ball of the foot.

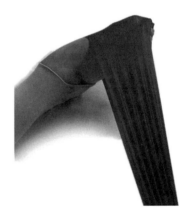

Exercise TB 3
DORSI FLEXION OF THE ANKLE

Support the working foot by resting it on the bent knee. Keep the foot pointed and apply pressure from the Theraband. Draw the foot toward the knee, working the muscles and tendon on the top of the foot. This strengthens the front of the ankle and the muscles on the outside (lateral side) of the calf to provide ankle support. Dorsi flexion is necessary when landing from a jump.

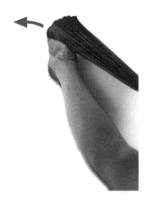

Exercise TB 4
EVERSION OF THE ANKLE

This exercise strengthens the muscles surrounding the ankle and the muscles on the lateral side (outside) of the calf, by working on straightening the foot from a turned-in or inverted position. This strengthening will help prevent ankle sprains as well as aiding in their speedy recovery. It also helps in stabilizing the ankle joint on flat surfaces or when rising onto the toe. For dancers, this strength is important in preventing "sickling" of the foot.

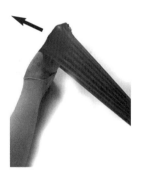

Exercise TB 5
INVERSION OF THE METATARSAL JOINT

This exercise will develop muscles in the front (anterior) part of the lower leg along the shin bone. This is necessary in stabilizing the muscles of the ankle and will help prevent rolling of the foot.

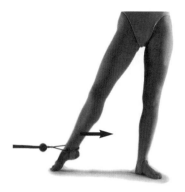

Exercise TB 6
ADDUCTION OF THE INNER THIGH

Place the rope end of the Theraband in a door at calf level and close the door with the loop on the other side of the door. This will hold the Theraband securely. This exercise strengthens the inner thigh muscles (adductors) of the working leg and, more important, the adductor muscles of the supporting leg. Turn out the working leg with the Theraband wrapped around the ankle, and draw the heel toward the supporting foot. The muscle that is actually worked is from the top of the inner thigh. As you release the foot, point it, keeping tension in the Theraband. For ballet dancers, this exercise develops the stability of the standing leg, helps build speed for *petite allegro*, and is necessary for *batterie* (*cabrioles, entrachat six, entrachat huit,* switching legs in double *tours,* etc.).

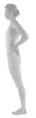

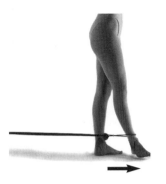

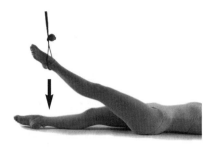

Exercise TB 7
FLEXION AND EXTENSION OF THE LEG WHILE USING OUTWARD ROTATION OF THE HIP JOINTS

This is another exercise to strengthen the inner thigh muscles of both legs. This helps greatly with the external rotation of the thigh (femur). If you feel any discomfort in the knee joint, bend the knee slightly. Start with both legs together and extend the working foot forward as far as possible, pointing the foot at the same time, then returning to the starting position.

Exercise TB 9
FLEXION TO EXTENSION ON THE BACK

Place the loop of the Theraband over the top of a door and shut the door so the loop is securely fastened. Lie on your back and place one foot in the handle of the Theraband. Keeping both legs turned out, draw the working leg down to the floor. This movement strengthens and tones the posterior (behind) part of the legs, including the gluteus (buttock) muscles. This strength is required for isolation from the hip joint and stability in the pelvic region (ballet dancers: for jumps and *adagios*).

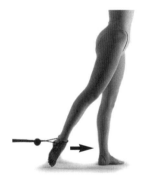

Exercise TB 8
HYPEREXTENSION TO EXTENSION

This exercise is designed to strengthen the front of the inner thigh. The resistance required to bring the leg from the hyperextended position (behind you) to the extended position (legs together) is helpful in working the muscles around, and especially in the front of, the hip socket. Perform the exercise without arching the back when the leg hyperextends (doing the B-Line will help a great deal).

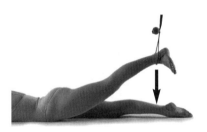

Exercise TB 10
PRONE HYPEREXTENSION TO EXTENSION

Lying on the stomach, do the B-Line, keep the hipbones flat on the floor, and externally rotate the legs. The resistance will create strength and tone in the front of the thighs.

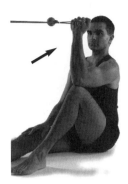

Exercise TB 11
BICEPS

Hold the handle and sit 3 to 4 feet away. Rest the working elbow on the bent knee. Draw the handle to the shoulder, stretching the Theraband. Resist the tension upon release. This should feel as if the middle of the forearm were drawing towards the bicep, rather than the hand toward the shoulder.

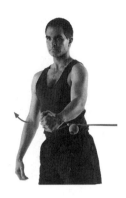

Exercise TB 13
PECTORALS

Stand at a 90-degree angle to a closed door, about 3 to 6 feet away, hold the handle, and with a slightly flexed (bent) elbow, draw the Theraband across the chest. Keep the elbow in a fixed position and do not rotate the upper body to move the arm farther.

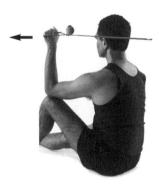

Exercise TB 12
TRICEPS

Sit on the floor with your back to a door about 3 to 4 feet away. Rest the working elbow on the bent knee and extend the arm to a fully extended position. Resist upon the release.

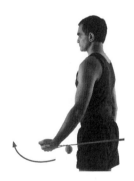

Exercise TB 14
PECTORALS AND DELTOIDS

Stand with your back to a door about 3 to 6 feet away. Hold the handle and keep the elbow in a flexed position. Draw the handle forward to the hip and then continue forward to shoulder level. Resist upon the return. Keep the upper body stable.

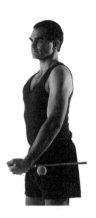

Exercise TB 15
LATISSIMUS DORSI

Stand at a 90-degree angle to a closed door, about 3 to 6 feet away. Hold the Theraband taut away from the body. Draw the Theraband to your side, pressing the arm to the floor. To better connect the lat, imagine you are squashing an orange under the armpit as you press the arm to your side. Resist upon the return.

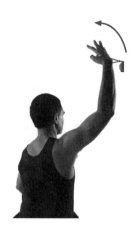

Exercise TB 17
OVERHEAD

Stand at a 90-degree angle to a closed door with the working arm extended to the ceiling and at about a 45-degree angle to the door. Keeping a slight bend in the elbow, extend the arm overhead away from the door. This exercise will work the shoulder muscles. If you feel any discomfort in the neck, stop the exercise.

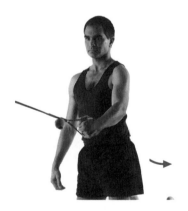

Exercise TB 16
BACK

Face a door about 3 to 6 feet away. With the arm extended forward at chest level, draw the handle parallel to the floor as far to the outside as possible. Keep the shoulders square to the door at all times. Imagine drawing the shoulder blades together; this will strengthen the rhomboid muscles between the shoulder blades.

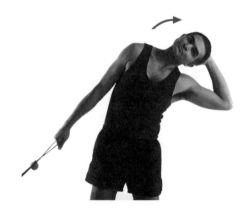

Exercise TB 18
SIDE STRETCH

Stand at a 90-degree angle to a closed door. With the Theraband secured to the bottom of the door, place your free hand on the side of the head, keeping the elbow open wide. Stretch to the side, extending through the tip of the elbow in an arc so the side does not crunch. Lift up and out of the hip as if stretching over a ball. Keep the hips firm and square. This is an important exercise for strengthening the side muscles (quadratus lumborum).

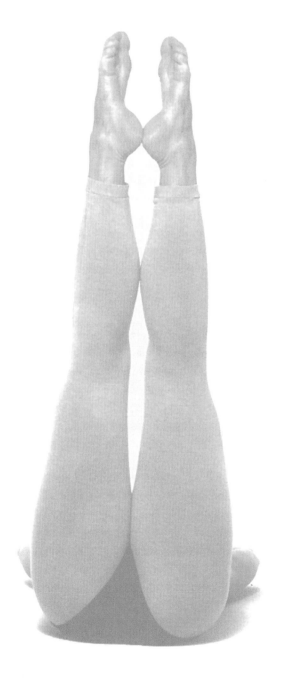

CHAPTER 12

Move Yourself out of Pain

Physical fitness can neither be acquired by wishful thinking nor by outright purchase. However, it can be gained through performing these (daily) exercises conceived for this purpose by the founder of Contrology® whose unique methods accomplish this desirable result by successfully counteracting the harmful, inherent conditions associated with modern civilization.

RETURN TO LIFE THROUGH CONTROLOGY®

The ultimate goal of any therapeutic or rehabilitation exercise program is to achieve pain-free movement. But many people who are in some pain, even though they have passed the acute stage of their problem, are still reluctant to move the areas of the body where they previously felt pain. This protective attitude toward the body can be detrimental in the long term to a person's well-being.

This mental protection of the physical structure inhibits recovery, rehabilitation, and progress to normal movement. Over time, an imbalance is created, which the body will accept as normal and which the mind, eventually, also accepts.

In this chapter we shall discuss general rehabilitation exercises for the various parts of the body, in cases where the condition is no longer in the acute phases and the treating practitioner has given permission for a post-acute exercise program.

It is important to realize that beginning an exercise program does not mean immediate relief. Even though some of the benefits may be immediate, while the mind is willing to achieve a normal lifestyle, the body is still physically weak.

Too often has it been reported that when the symptoms of pain have disappeared for some minutes, the patient assumes that the condition is fixed and he is able to return to normal activity.

Sadly, this is far from the truth. The feeling of well-being may only be temporary. Although the injury may have taken only a matter of seconds to inflict, it may take months to repair. This can be very frustrating to the individual who is on a mission to be better in the shortest time possible. Remember, it was the tortoise who won the race!

The exercise rehabilitation process has two main objectives:

1. To reduce the recovery time for each episode in which the injured area is affected by overexertion, either intentionally or accidentally.

2. To substantially strengthen the area.

Say, for example, an individual has lower back pain. She has not begun any exercise program; however, when her back "goes out," it takes two days for the pain to diminish. Starting a personalized exercise program does not mean the problem will be solved overnight. However, if the back goes out again, the program, if effectively implemented, should reduce the recovery time (from two days to possibly only a few hours.) Each subsequent time the back goes out, the recovery time should be shorter than the last. As muscular stability is achieved, this recovery time should continue to reduce.

CASE STUDY

A middle-aged man of slightly larger-than-average build had dislocated his right shoulder eight times in the previous two years. Previous rehabilitation exercises involved raising weights, in a standing position, up to shoulder level and no higher.

When asked about the mobility of the joint, the patient responded that he was only able to raise the arm to shoulder height and would not attempt to raise it any higher (possibly for fear of another dislocation), even without weights.

The last dislocation had occurred eight months previously; the patient was convinced that his current range of movement was set for all time.

After doing a series of arm-weight exercises while lying supine on a narrow bench (lifting nothing above shoulder height), the client was then told to lie face-down. He was asked to raise the arms out to the sides to bench level and return to the starting position. This was well within the client's perceived comfort zone, and he completed several repetitions easily.

After doing several of these movements, the client was then asked to raise the left arm to the left ear and the right arm to the right hip, and then to alternate the movement (similar to a marching movement). He accomplished this without any effort or fear. When he raised the right arm to the ear for the third time, the client was asked to hold the position and to imagine that he was in an upright position. This came as quite a surprise to the client, as the arm was above head height. He was then asked to stand and repeat the movement without fear. Once his fear had been overcome, the rehabilitation of the shoulder was more effective, with faster results.

There may be setbacks along the way, when the patient will feel more pain. One reason for this is that, as the program progresses, the imbalance already accentuated in the individual because of the injury is exacerbated. This happens because the stronger muscles continue to dominate the movement, while the weaker muscles tend initially to lag behind. This produces further imbalances as the strong muscles "pull" the structure out of alignment. This situation is usually indicated by the fact that discomfort occurs and remains no matter what stretches are prescribed to alleviate it. This discomfort is easily remedied by gentle manipulation to "realign" the problem area, after which and the exercise program can be continued. (Please consult your physical therapist if this occurs.)

When attending these realignment sessions with a qualified practitioner, it is important to remember that you should do no exercises for at least 24 to 36 hours after the treatment in order for it to settle into the muscular system.

As the recovery time approaches zero, the true strengthening phase of the program can begin. Keep in mind the guidelines mentioned in Chapter 3, "Joint Strains."

THE CONDITIONS AND THE EXERCISES THAT BRING RELIEF

In the descriptions of the conditions that follow, the exercises have been numbered to assist in quick reference. If the exercise is new, a description is included.

The Ankles and Feet

For weak ankles and feet, including pronation, supination, flat feet, and weak toes:

All ankle Theraband work, TB 1 to TB 5

Plus *Exercises 8-1, 8-2*   Calf Stretches

The Knee

For weak knee joints, including chondromalacia of the patella and Patella Tracking Syndrome:

Exercises 8-1, 8-2	Calf Stretches
Exercises 26-1, 26-2, 26-3	Ankle Weights

Plus Theraband:

Exercise TB 6	Adduction of the Inner Thigh
Exercise TB 8	Hyperextension to Extension

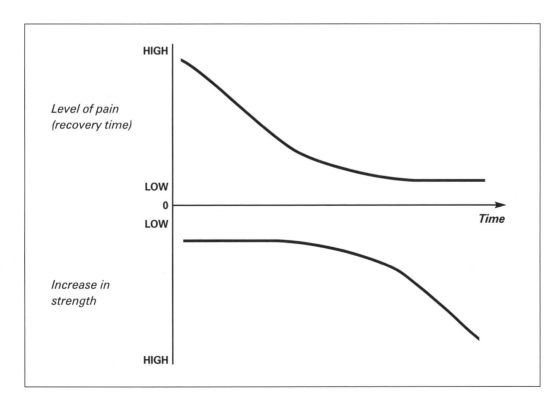

Exercise TB 7	Flexion and Extension of the Leg while Using Outward Rotation of the Hip Joints

The Hip Joint

Theraband work Exercise TB 6 to TB 10

Plus

Exercise 70	Helicopter Hundreds
Exercise 20	Single Leg Stretch
Exercise 22	Single Leg Circles 1
Exercise 62	Pendulum
Exercise 49	Side Kick 1
Exercise 56	Side Kick 2
Exercises 26-1, 26-2, 26-3	Ankle Weights
Exercise 72	Standing Side Stretches: Basic

The Back

Lower back pain is one of the most common complaints in Western society. The complaints range from minor backache, which can be fixed with massage, manipulation, or anti-inflammatory drugs, to more serious cases, such as disc protrusions and spondylolisthesis (the forward slippage of one vertebra onto another), to those that require surgery.

Clearly graduated exercise programs are the best long-term management for lower back pain. These take the form of gradual stretching and strengthening.

It is often more important to know what *not* to do, as these movements can set back the program and irritate the condition.

Listed below are some of the movements to avoid for certain conditions, followed by simple routines to practice. For all back problems, the start stretches, hamstring stretches, and thigh stretches should be done unless there are contraindications to the stretches.

The next three stretches are to be completed in all cases unless indications are that they are impossible to achieve even in the mildest form.

Exercises 3 to 6a	The Start Stretches
Exercises 9-1, 9-2	Hamstring Stretches

Exercises 11 to 13	Thigh Stretches

(lying, standing, or kneeling, depending on the tightness of the thighs)

For posterior disc bulges, avoid any forward flexion exercises. Instead, do the following:

Exercise 24	Stomach Stretch
Exercise 25	The Perfect Abdominal Curl
Exercise 20	Single Leg Stretch
Exercise 21	Double Leg Stretch: Basic
Exercise 22	Single Leg Circles 1
Exercise 18	The Hundreds: Basic

For one-sided sciatic problems, avoid exercises that contract the lower back muscles on the side where the sciatic pain is located. Stretch the tight side. Follow the exercises below, placing particular emphasis on repeating twice as many sets on the tight side of the back:

Exercise 7	Spiral Stretch
Exercise 44	Spine Rotation (Spine Twist)
Exercise 25	The Perfect Abdominal Curl
Exercise 38	Single Leg Stretch with Rotation: Criss-Cross
Exercise 50-1	Side Leg Lifts
Exercise 21	Double Leg Stretch: Basic
Exercise 43	Swimming
Exercise 72	Standing Side Stretches: Basic

If you have sciatic pain down both legs, avoid hyperextending the lower back. Follow these exercises:

Exercise 51	Pelvic Curl
Exercise 73	Cat Stretch

If you have scoliosis, avoid leaning the torso to the short side of the curve. The exercise program is the same as that for one-sided sciatic pain.

If you have lumbar lordosis, avoid arching the back in that area. Follow these exercises:

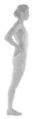

Exercise 2	Standing Spine Roll
Exercise 45	Spine Stretch
Exercise 18	The Hundreds: Basic
Exercise 32	Coordination
Exercise 20	Single Leg Stretch
Exercise 21	Double Leg Stretch: Basic
Exercise 22	Single Leg Circles 1
Exercise 25	The Perfect Abdominal Curl
Exercise 76	Oblique Curls
Exercise 51	Pelvic Curl
Exercise 73	Cat Stretch
Exercise 44	Spine Rotation (Spine Twist)
Exercise 1	Resting Position

If you have cervical lordosis, lie on the floor and place the arms at shoulder height away from the body with the palms facing up. Place a small, soft cushion under the arch of the neck and, breathing out, press the neck onto the cushion, without rounding the shoulders.

Also do this exercise:

Exercise 78	Neck Stretches

In addition, do the following: Sitting upright, interlock the fingers behind the head. Stretch the chin to the chest and, breathing out, resist with the hands as you try to stretch the *back* of the neck to the ceiling. Do not lift from the top of the head. Press the shoulder blades to the floor. Repeat ten times.

The Shoulders

For shoulder problems and kyphosis (middle/upper thoracic spine), avoid forward flexion of the back in that area.

Follow these exercises (always with a cushion under the forehead to support the neck in a stretched position):

Exercise 39	Stomach Stretch: Alternating Arms and Legs
Exercise 43	Swimming
Exercise 30	The Pole

Exercises 28-1 to 28-4	Arm Weights
Exercises 29-1, 29-2	Arm Swings
Exercise 78	Neck Stretches

The following basic routine is suggested for most low-grade lower back pain:

Exercise 45	Spine Stretch
Exercise 23	Side to Side
Exercise 18	The Hundreds: Basic
Exercise 32	Coordination
Exercise 21	Double Leg Stretch: Basic
Exercise 20	Single Leg Stretch
Exercise 25	The Perfect Abdominal Curl
Exercise 24	Stomach Stretch
Exercise 51	Pelvic Curl
Exercise 44	Spine Rotation (Spine Twist)
Exercise 73	Cat Stretch

As an exercise becomes less of a challenge, progress to the next version of the exercise, keeping in mind all the finer points of the exercise listed under Key Points and Care.

THE CHALLENGE

To help you progress from the basic routine, I have compiled a list of exercises in progressive order. You should begin with Stage I and continue in order through Stage VI. If you are unable to complete perfectly one of the exercises in a stage, you should not attempt to proceed to the next stage.

The challenge is to control the manner in which you perform the routine, not how many exercises you can do in the shortest period of time.

The basic routine is adequate for beginners of any age, including children (if your child is experiencing a growth spurt, first check with your medical practitioner or a qualified Pilates practitioner).

Although Pilates' method has become widely known as an aid in rehabilitating people with many types of injuries and conditions, the Challenge routines described here do not take into account specific injuries or unusual conditions.

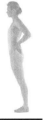

Therefore, you should not attempt them without first consulting a qualified Pilates practitioner.

For the convenience of those wishing to record their progress during the various stages of the program, I have included charts covering six stages of the Method. Complete one stage at a time. Do the exercises three times a week (more if you wish). In the box for each exercise and date, state the level of effort or challenge you felt for the exercise. For example, the following chart shows that on Monday the standing spine roll required an effort of 7 out of 10. If the challenge falls below 5 out of 10 on the effort scale, then progress to a harder version of the exercise. If there isn't a harder version, then progress to a different but similar exercise that poses a challenge. When you can do 75 percent of the exercises in a stage with ease, move on to the next stage, but regularly go back to the exercises you found challenging until you are comfortable with them. Photocopy the charts to add further weeks to the program, if you wish.

Good luck! You will be glad you took the opportunity, and I am pleased to have been able to present you the possibility to change your life in a positive way.

Basic Routine

| *Exercise 2* | Standing Spine Roll |
| *Exercises 3 to 6a* | The Start Stretches |

Exercise 9-1	Hamstring Stretch: Basic
Exercise 12	Thigh Stretch 2: Standing
Exercise 45	Spine Stretch
Exercise 50-1	Side Leg Lifts
Exercise 16	Preparation with Cushions
Exercise 18	The Hundreds: Basic
Exercise 32	Coordination
Exercise 20	Single Leg Stretch
Exercise 21	Double Leg Stretch: Basic
Exercise 25	The Perfect Abdominal Curl
Exercise 73	Cat Stretch
Exercise 28-1	Opening Arms
Exercises 29-1, 29-2	Arm Swings
Exercise 1	Resting Position

Stage I

Exercise 2	Standing Spine Roll
Exercises 3 to 6a	The Start Stretches
Exercise 10	Hamstring Stretch 3
Exercise 13	Thigh Stretch 3: Kneeling
Exercise 45	Spine Stretch

BASIC ROUTINE EXERCISE CHART

EXERCISE	WEEK 1			WEEK 2			WEEK 3			WEEK 4		
PROGRAM DATE: 6/22/00	M	W	F	M	W	F	M	W	F	M	W	F
#2 Standing Spine Roll	7	6	4									
#3 to 6a The Start Stretches	7	6	7									
#9-1 Hamstring Stretch: Basic	8	8	7									
#12 Thigh Stretch 2: Standing	9	8	7									
#45 Spine Stretch	7	7	6									
#50-1 Side Leg Lifts	8	8	7									
#16 Preparation with Cushions	8	7	6									
#18 The Hundreds: Basic	8	8	8									
#32 Coordination	8	7	8									
#20 Single Leg Stretch	6	6	6									
#21 Double Leg Stretch: Basic	8	7	8									
#25 The Perfect Abdominal Curl	8	8	8									
#73 Cat Stretch	6	6	6									
#28-1 Opening Arms	8	7	7									
#29-1, 29-2 Arm Swings	6	6	6									
#1 Resting Position	8	7										

Exercise 20	Single Leg Stretch	*Exercise 59*	Control Balance
Exercise 36	Double Leg Stretch 2: Lowering and Raising	*Exercise 65*	Scissors
		Exercise 74	Rocking
Exercise 47-2	Corkscrew 2: Advanced	*Exercise 49*	Side Kick 1
Exercise 46	Open Leg Rocker	*Exercise 28*	Arm Weights: All Supine Routines
Exercise 34	The Roll-Over (or Spine Roll)	*Exercise 27*	Back of the Thigh: Hamstring/Buttocks
Exercise 61	Roll-Over: Bent Legs	*Exercises 29-1, 29-2*	Arm Swings
Exercise 53-1	Teaser 1: Basic	*Exercise 72*	Standing Side Stretches: Basic
Exercise 54	Leg Pull Front		
Exercise 55	Leg Pull Back		
Exercise 64	Jackknife	**Stage VI**	
Exercise 59	Control Balance		
Exercise 28	Arm Weights: All Supine Routines	*Exercises 3 to 6a*	The Start Stretches
		Exercise 8-2	Alternating Calf Stretches
Exercise 26-1	Ankle Weights: Outer Thigh (Abductor)	*Exercise 10*	Hamstring Stretch 3
Exercises 29-1, 29-2	Arm Swings	*Exercise 13*	Thigh Stretch 3: Kneeling
Exercise 30	The Pole	*Exercise 33*	The Roll-Up
Exercise 72	Standing Side Stretches: Basic	*Exercise 25*	The Perfect Abdominal Curl
		Exercise 35	Single Leg Circles
Stage V		*Exercise 38*	Single Leg Stretch with Rotation: Criss-Cross
Exercises 3 to 6a	The Start Stretches	*Exercise 36*	Double Leg Stretch 2: (Variation)
Exercise 9-2	Hamstring Stretch 2	*Exercise 34*	The Roll-Over (or Spine Roll)
Exercise 13	Thigh Stretch 3: Kneeling	*Exercise 61*	Roll-Over: Bent Legs
Exercise 60	The Hundreds: Lower and Raise	*Exercise 44*	Spine Rotation (Spine Twist)
Exercise 25	The Perfect Abdominal Curl	*Exercise 48*	The Saw
Exercise 76	Oblique Curls	*Exercise 47-2*	Corkscrew 2: Advanced
Exercise 63	Neck Pull	*Exercise 42-1*	Swan Dive 2 (Rocking Press-Up 2)
Exercise 36	Double Leg Stretch 2: Lowering and Raising	*Exercise 53-3*	Teaser 3
Exercise 38	Single Leg Stretch with Rotation: Criss-Cross	*Exercise 65*	Scissors
		Exercise 66	Bicycle
Exercise 47-2	Corkscrew 2: Advanced	*Exercise 1*	Resting Position
Exercise 62	Pendulum	*Exercise 54*	Leg Pull Front
Exercise 69	Hip Circles	*Exercise 55*	Leg Pull Back
Exercise 61	Roll-Over: Bent Legs	*Exercise 56*	Side Kick 2
Exercise 53-2	Teaser 2	*Exercise 57*	Boomerang
Exercise 54	Leg Pull Front	*Exercise 59*	Control Balance
Exercise 58	Seal	*Exercise 75-1*	Twist 1
Exercise 42-1	Swan Dive 2 (Rocking Press-Up 2)	*Exercise 28-4*	Arm Circles
		Exercise 72	Standing Side Stretches: Basic
Exercise 68-1	Can-Can Extension		

Exercise 71	Lying Torso Stretch
Exercises 29-1, 29-2	Arm Swings
Exercise 30	The Pole

STUDIO-BASED PROGRAMS

Beyond the floor routines, there are the studio-based programs. It is always advisable to check to ensure that the studio you wish to attend is a registered, certified studio with an established reputation. The studio programs are by appointment and are able to give you the full benefit of all Joe Pilates' work. Under the watchful eye of an instructor, you will be guided through programs suited to your strengths and weaknesses.

Within the studio environment, there are a variety of pieces of equipment with curious names such as the Universal Reformer®, the Cadillac®, the Wunda Chair®, and the Pedi-Pul®. The use of specialized equipment challenges your body to a different level. This is not to diminish the importance of the floor routines. As a stand-alone program, the floor routines can be done in any place at any time—a considerable advantage over the equipment-based routines.

CONCLUSION

When putting Joseph Pilates' body control techniques to work, you will undoubtedly notice some changes quite soon. To get the most from the program, however, it is also important to be aware of the response your body and muscles are feeding back to you. When you feel you have mastered a program adequately, remain with that program for an additional week to consolidate the connection of the mind and the body on those movements.

This may feel akin to watching a film for the second time and noticing small, but important, aspects that you were unaware of the first time. If one small aspect of the film were missing, it would not dramatically change the overall message or content of the film. However, if a large section or the total of these small parts were missing, the film would give the viewer a totally different message! So it is with the Pilates work. You, as the viewer, will gradually improve your perception and control over the smaller, once seemingly insignificant, details of the movements. As the parts fuse together to become the whole, the body will regain lost perceptions. The mind and body will work in unison, and the sense of well-being, both mental and physical, will produce an emotional enthusiasm that your body has not felt for some time—if ever!

I have attempted to be as precise as possible in all the descriptions of the movements. Focus on each of them. As you become more proficient at the routines, review them after a month, even when you have progressed to the next stage. Scrutinize the procedure to see if you have incorporated every aspect into the movement so that your mind and body are getting the full, clear message.

As the viewer, you will not only see the benefits of what Pilates' exercises can do for your body; you will become so involved in the film that you will also feel the reality from deep within.

REFERENCES

Arnheim, Daniel. *Modern Principles of Athletic Training*. St. Louis, MO: Times Mirror, 1989.

Eisen, G., and Freidman, R. *The Pilates Method of Mental and Physical Conditioning*. New York: Warner, 1980 (out of print).

Fitt, S. S. *Dance Kinesiology*. New York: Schirmer Books, 1988.

Howse, J., and Hancock, S. *Dance Technique and Injury Prevention*. London: A & C Black, 1998.

Kapandji, I. A. *The Physiology of the Joints*. Edinburgh: Churchill Livingston, 1974.

Kendall, F. P., and McCreary, E. K. *Muscles Testing and Function*. Baltimore, MD: Williams & Wilkins, 1993.

Kisner, C., and Colby, L. A. *Therapeutic Exercise*. Philadelphia, PA: F. A. Davis, 1988.

Peterson, L., and Renstrom, P. *Sports Injuries*. Auckland, New Zealand: Methuen, 1988.

Ryan, A. J., and Stephens, R. E. *Dance Medicine*. Chicago: Pluribus Press, 1987.

Winter Griffith, H. *Sports Injuries*. Tucson, AZ: The Body Press, 1986.

STUDIOS TEACHING THE TECHNIQUES OF JOSEPH H. PILATES

United States

Physicalmind Institute
1807 2nd St., Suites 15 and 40
Santa Fe NM 87505
Tel: (505) 988-1990 or toll free (800) 505-1990

Bodyscapes
Angela Sundberg
7835 E. Gelding Dr.
Scottsdale AZ 85260
Tel: (480) 991-8811

Bodyline Fitness Studio
Maria Leone-Seid
367 South Doheny Dr.
Beverly Hills CA 90211
Tel: (310) 274-2716

Live Art Studios
Siri Galliano
1100 South Beverly Dr., Suite 208
Beverly Hills CA 90035
Tel: (310) 277-9536

Celebrate Life
JoEllyn Musser
24725 Pennsylvania Ave., #C-20
Lomita CA 90717
Tel: (310) 530-7881

ShapeShift Studio
Nancy Coleman
1820 S. Catalina Ave., Suite 105
Redondo Beach CA 90277
Tel: (310) 543-2327

ShapeShift Studio–Palos Verdes
James Hume
627 Silver Spur Rd.–300C
Rolling Hills Estates CA 90274
Tel: (310) 544-4355

Balance Fitness Studio
Michele Vaughan-Shannon
1626A Union St.
San Francisco CA 94123
Tel: (415) 441-6488

Dewild Studio
Astrid de Wild
330 E. Canon Perdido St., Suite D
Santa Barbara CA 93101
Tel: (805) 564-3454

Susan Lonergan
13364 Contour Dr.
Sherman Oaks CA 91423
Tel: (818) 905-6856

MeJo Wiggin
(phone for location)
Central Greenwich CT
Tel: (203) 629-3743

Body in Balance
Fran Ahrens
50 South Washington
Hinsdale IL 60521
Tel: (630) 655-9922 or toll free (877) 655-9923

The Body Fit Conditioning Studio
Leslie Kubas
9404 W. 83rd St.
Overland Park KS 66204
Tel: (913) 648-0990

SOMA
Ily Shofestall
585 Main St., Suite 3
Rockland ME 04841
Tel: (207) 596-6177

New Millennium Wellness
Barbara O'Shea
2409 Old Mill Rd.
Spring Lake Heights NJ 07762
Tel: (732) 282-0600

Anthony Rabara Studio
Anthony Rabara
392 Wall St.
Princeton NJ 08540
Tel: (609) 921-7990

Tribeca Bodyworks
Alycea Ungaro
117 Duane St.
New York NY 10013
Tel: (212) 625-0777

Body Works
Tami Casey and Leslie Braverman
5319 SW Westgate Dr., #224
Portland OR 97221
Tel: (503) 292-3800

Elite Fitness
Elizabeth Morrissey
2 N. Collingwood Dr.
Pittsburg PA 15215
Tel: (412) 781-3443

Body Precision Inc.
Beth Downey
28 Garrett Ave.
Rosemont PA 19010
Tel: (610) 520-BRIT (520-2748)

Wendy LeBlanc-Arbuckle
700 Zennia
Austin TX 78757
Tel: (512) 467-8009

Good Body's (Formerly Glenn Studio Inc.)
Colleen Glenn
5301 West Lovers Ln., #114
Dallas TX 75209
Tel: (214) 351-9931

The Physical Therapy Center of Seattle
413 Fairview Ave. N.
Seattle WA 98109
Tel: (206) 405-3560

Canada

Go Physiotherapy
Joanna Spellar
100 James St. S.
Hamilton, Ontario L8P 2Z2
Canada
Tel: (905) 528-5847

Fitness and Rehabilitation Studio Inc.
Monique Haziza
#4–302 West 2nd Ave.
Vancouver V5Y 1C8
Canada
Tel: (604) 875-0404

Australia

For inquiries on videos, equipment, training, or registering your studio on the Internet, please contact:

The Pilates Institute of Australasia
PO Box 1046
North Sydney NSW 2059
Australia
Tel: +612-9267-8223
Fax: +612-9267-8226
Internet: www.pilates.net

BASIC ROUTINE EXERCISE CHART

EXERCISE	WEEK 1			WEEK 2			WEEK 3			WEEK 4			WEEK 5			WEEK 6			WEEK 7		
PROGRAM DATE: / /	M	W	F	M	W	F	M	W	F	M	W	F	M	W	F	M	W	F	M	W	F
#2 Standing Spine Roll																					
#3 to 6a The Start Stretches																					
#9-1 Hamstring Stretch: Basic																					
#12 Thigh Stretch 2: Standing																					
#45 Spine Stretch																					
#50-1 Side Leg Lifts																					
#16 Preparation with Cushions																					
#18 The Hundreds: Basic																					
#32 Coordination																					
#20 Single Leg Stretch																					
#21 Double Leg Stretch: Basic																					
#25 The Perfect Abdominal Curl																					
#73 Cat Stretch																					
#28-1 Opening Arms																					
#29-1, 29-2 Arm Swings																					
#1 Resting Position																					

STAGE I EXERCISE CHART

EXERCISE	WEEK 1			WEEK 2			WEEK 3			WEEK 4			WEEK 5			WEEK 6			WEEK 7		
PROGRAM DATE: /	M	W	F	M	W	F	M	W	F	M	W	F	M	W	F	M	W	F	M	W	F
#2 Standing Spine Roll																					
#3 to 6a The Start Stretches																					
#10 Hamstring Stretch 3																					
#13 Thigh Stretch 3: Kneeling																					
#45 Spine Stretch																					
#44 Spine Rotation (Spine Twist)																					
#48 The Saw																					
#16 Preparation with Cushions																					
#19-1 The Hundreds: Intermediate																					
#25 The Perfect Abdominal Curl																					
#76 Oblique Curls																					
#20 Single Leg Stretch																					
#21 Double Leg Stretch: Basic																					
#33 The Roll-Up																					
#37 Rolling																					
#47 Corkscrew: Basic																					
#24 Stomach Stretch																					
#28-1, 28-2 Opening Arms: Alternating																					
#26-1, 26-2 Ankle Weights																					
#29-1, 29-2 Arm Swings																					
#30 The Pole																					

STAGE II EXERCISE CHART

EXERCISE	WEEK 1			WEEK 2			WEEK 3			WEEK 4			WEEK 5			WEEK 6			WEEK 7		
PROGRAM DATE: / /	M	W	F	M	W	F	M	W	F	M	W	F	M	W	F	M	W	F	M	W	F
#3 to 6a The Start Stretches																					
#9-2 Hamstring Stretch 2																					
#13 Thigh Stretch 3: Kneeling																					
#76 Oblique Curls																					
#23 Side to Side																					
#31 The Hundreds: Alternating Legs																					
#47 Corkscrew: Basic																					
#62 Pendulum																					
#33 The Roll-Up																					
#46 Open Leg Rocker																					
#20 Single Leg Stretch																					
#36 Double Leg Stretch 2																					
#43 Swimming																					
#49 Side Kick 1																					
#28 Arm Weights: All Supine Routines																					
#29-1, 29-2 Arm Swings																					
#30 The Pole																					
#72 Standing Side Stretches: Basic																					

STAGE III EXERCISE CHART

EXERCISE	WEEK 1			WEEK 2			WEEK 3			WEEK 4			WEEK 5			WEEK 6			WEEK 7		
PROGRAM DATE: / /	M	W	F	M	W	F	M	W	F	M	W	F	M	W	F	M	W	F	M	W	F
#3 to 6a The Start Stretches																					
#9-2 Hamstring Stretch 2																					
#13 Thigh Stretch 3: Kneeling																					
#23 Side to Side																					
#47-1 Corkscrew 1: Intermediate																					
#62 Pendulum																					
#63 Neck Pull																					
#76 Oblique Curls																					
#38 Single Leg Stretch with Rotation																					
#60 The Hundreds: Lower and Raise																					
#36 Double Leg Stretch 2																					
#34 The Roll Over (or Spine Roll)																					
#69 Hip Circles																					
#64 Jackknife																					
#58 Seal																					
#53-1 Teaser 1: Basic																					
#40 Single Leg Kick																					
#28 Arm Weights: All Supine Routines																					
#29-1, 29-2 Arm Swings																					
#72 Standing Side Stretches: Basic																					
#30 The Pole																					

STAGE IV EXERCISE CHART

EXERCISE	WEEK 1			WEEK 2			WEEK 3			WEEK 4			WEEK 5			WEEK 6			WEEK 7		
PROGRAM DATE: / /	M	W	F	M	W	F	M	W	F	M	W	F	M	W	F	M	W	F	M	W	F
#3 to 6a The Start Stretches																					
#9-2 Hamstring Stretch 2																					
#13 Thigh Stretch 3: Kneeling																					
#31 The Hundreds: Alternating Legs																					
#25 The Perfect Abdominal Curl																					
#76 Oblique Curls																					
#63 Neck Pull																					
#20 Single Leg Stretch																					
#36 Double Leg Stretch 2																					
#47-2 Corkscrew 2: Advanced																					
#46 Open Leg Rocker																					
#34 The Roll-Over (or Spine Roll)																					
#61 Roll-Over: Bent Legs																					
#53-1 Teaser 1: Basic																					
#54 Leg Pull Front																					
#55 Leg Pull Back																					
#64 Jackknife																					
#59 Control Balance																					
#28 Arm Weights: All Supine Routines																					
#26-1 Ankle Weights: Outer Thigh																					
#29-1, 29-2 Arm Swings																					
#30 The Pole																					
#72 Standing Side Stretches: Basic																					

STAGE V EXERCISE CHART

EXERCISE	WEEK 1			WEEK 2			WEEK 3			WEEK 4			WEEK 5			WEEK 6			WEEK 7		
PROGRAM DATE: / /	M	W	F	M	W	F	M	W	F	M	W	F	M	W	F	M	W	F	M	W	F
#3 to 6a The Start Stretches																					
#9-2 Hamstring Stretch 2																					
#13 Thigh Stretch 3: Kneeling																					
#60 The Hundreds: Lower and Raise																					
#25 The Perfect Abdominal Curl																					
#76 Oblique Curls																					
#63 Neck Pull																					
#36 Double Leg Stretch 2																					
#38 Single Leg Stretch with Rotation																					
#47-2 Corkscrew 2: Advanced																					
#62 Pendulum																					
#69 Hip Circles																					
#61 Roll-Over: Bent Legs																					
#53-2 Teaser 2																					
#54 Leg Pull Front																					
#58 Seal																					
#42-1 Swan Dive 2																					
#68-1 Can Can Extension																					
#59 Control Balance																					
#65 Scissors																					
#74 Rocking																					
#49 Side Kick 1																					
#28 Arm Weights: All Supine Routines																					
#27 Back of the Thigh																					
#29-1, 29-2 Arm Swings																					
#72-1 Standing Side Stretches: Basic																					

STAGE VI EXERCISE CHART

EXERCISE	WEEK 1			WEEK 2			WEEK 3			WEEK 4			WEEK 5			WEEK 6			WEEK 7		
PROGRAM DATE: / /	M	W	F	M	W	F	M	W	F	M	W	F	M	W	F	M	W	F	M	W	F
#3 to 6a The Start Stretches																					
#8-2 Alternating Calf Stretches																					
#10 Hamstrings Stretch 3																					
#13 Thigh Stretch 3: Kneeling																					
#33 The Roll-Up																					
#25 The Perfect Abdominal Curl																					
#35 Single Leg Circles																					
#38 Single Leg Stretch with Rotation																					
#36 Double Leg Stretch 2 (Variation)																					
#34 The Roll Over (or Spine Roll)																					
#61 Roll Over: Bent Legs																					
#44 Spine Rotation (Spine Twist)																					
#48 The Saw																					
#47-2 Corkscrew 2: Advanced																					
#42-1 Swan Dive 2																					
#53-3 Teaser 3																					
#65 Scissors																					
#66 Bicycle																					
#1 Resting Position																					
#54 Leg Pull Front																					
#55 Leg Pull Back																					
#56 Side Kick 2																					
#57 Boomerang																					
#59 Control Balance																					
#75-1 Twist 1																					
#28-4 Arm Circles																					
#72 Standing Side Stretches: Basic																					
#71 Lying Torso Stretch																					
#29-1, 29-2 Arm Swings																					
#30 The Pole																					

EXERCISE CHART

EXERCISE	WEEK 1			WEEK 2			WEEK 3			WEEK 4			WEEK 5			WEEK 6			WEEK 7		
	M	W	F	M	W	F	M	W	F	M	W	F	M	W	F	M	W	F	M	W	F
PROGRAM DATE: / /																					

EXERCISE CHART

EXERCISE	PROGRAM DATE: / /	WEEK 1			WEEK 2			WEEK 3			WEEK 4			WEEK 5			WEEK 6			WEEK 7		
		M	W	F	M	W	F	M	W	F	M	W	F	M	W	F	M	W	F	M	W	F

EXERCISE CHART

EXERCISE	WEEK 1			WEEK 2			WEEK 3			WEEK 4			WEEK 5			WEEK 6			WEEK 7		
PROGRAM DATE: / /	M	W	F	M	W	F	M	W	F	M	W	F	M	W	F	M	W	F	M	W	F

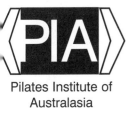

Pilates Institute of
Australasia

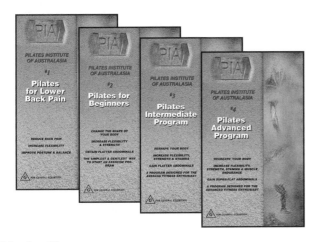

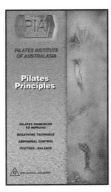

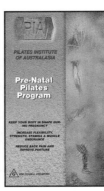

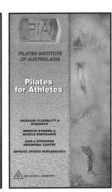

Shipping Charges
ONE VIDEO ONLY:

	Air Mail	Econ. Air	Surface
USA/CANADA	$13.50	$11.00	$10.00

COMPLETE SET OF VIDEOS 1–4:

	Air Mail	Econ. Air	Surface
USA/CANADA	$27.75	$21.50	$19.00

Add $8 for each additional video ordered. Orders will be shipped within 10 days of availability. Please allow 2 weeks air, 3 weeks economy air and 3 months surface for delivery.

- -

Name: _____

Address: _____

Zip Code: _____ State: _____ Country: _____

Telephone: _____ Fax: _____ Email: _____

Please send me...

☐ **1. Pilates for Lower Back Pain** for $29.95 + s&h ☐ **2. Pilates—for Beginners** for $29.95 + s&h

☐ **3. Pilates—Intermediate Program** for $29.95 + s&h ☐ **4. Pilates—Advanced Program** for $29.95 + s&h

OR

☐ **The complete set of videos 1–4** for only $99.95 p&h

☐ **Pilates Principles** for $29.95 + s&h ☐ **Pre-natal Pilates Program** for $39.95 + s&h

☐ **Pilates for Athletes** for $39.95 + s&h

Payment details...(For orders outside Australia, only credit card payments are accepted)

☐ Check ☐ Money Order Amount: $ _____ Shipping: $ _____

☐ Credit Card Amount: $ _____ ☐ Bankcard ☐ Visa ☐ MasterCard

Card #: _____ Expiration Date: _____

Name on Card: _____ Signature on Card: _____

Send completed form plus payment to: **Pilates Institute of Australasia (PIA), PO Box 1046, North Sydney NSW 2059, Australia or Fax: (+612) 9267 8226.**
If you have any queries, call the Pilates Institute of Australasia at Tel: (+612) 9267 8223; email: info@pilates.net or purchase online from: www.pilates.net

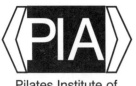

Pilates Institute of Australasia

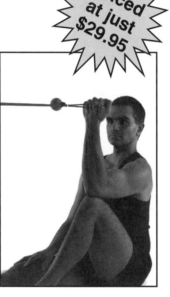
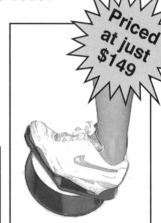
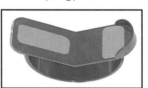

Order Other Hunter House Health and Fitness books

TREAT YOUR BACK WITHOUT SURGERY:
The Best Non-Surgical Alternatives for Eliminating Back and Neck Pain

by Stephen Hochschuler, M.D.,and Bob Reznik

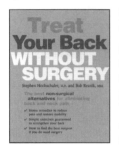

Eighty percent of back pain sufferers can get well without surgery. Be one of them! From the authors of *Back in Shape,* this new guide discusses a range of non-surgical techniques — from Tai Chi and massage therapy to chiropractic treatment and acupuncture — as well as exercise plans, diet and stress management techniques, and tips to ease everyday pain. Because surgery is sometimes necessary, you'll also get advice on how to find the best surgeon and what questions to ask.

224 pages ... 52 illus. ... Paperback $14.95

THE PLEASURE PRESCRIPTION: To Love, to Work, to Play—Life in the Balance
by Paul Pearsall, Ph.D.
New York Times Bestseller!

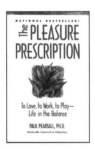

This bestselling book is a prescription for stressed-out lives. Dr. Pearsall maintains that contentment, wellness, and long life can be found by devoting time to family, helping others, and slowing down to savor life's pleasures. Pearsall's unique approach draws from Polynesian wisdom and his own 25 years of psychological and medical research. For readers who want to discover a way of life that promotes healthy values and living, *The Pleasure Prescription* provides the answers.

288 pages ... Paperback $13.95 ... Hard Cover $23.95

PEAK PERFORMANCE FITNESS: Maximizing Your Fitness Potential Without Injury or Strain
by Jennifer Rhodes, M.S.P.T. Foreword by Joan E. Edelstein

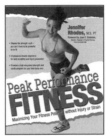

Jennifer Rhodes looks at the body as an integrated system and offers a step-by-step plan for developing cardiovascular capacity, strength, and flexibility. In a friendly, vibrant style she discusses the purpose of each exercise and how it works to improve the body's overall functioning. She gives real-life success stories of how her approach has helped clients, while detailed photographs and anatomical drawings illustrate the exercises. If you are serious about long-term health and want to get to your best body ever, this book will help you redefine the way you exercise and move.

160 pages ... 46 b/w photos ... 31 illus...Paperback ... $14.95

WRITE YOUR OWN PLEASURE PRESCRIPTION:
60 ways to Create Balance and Joy in Your Life
by Paul Pearsall, Ph.D.

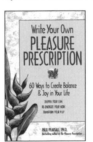

After the author appeared on The Montel Williams Show, *The Pleasure Prescription* rocketed to the top of the bestseller lists. Its message of finding and giving pleasure by reducing stress and cultivating harmony appealed to readers everywhere. A sequel to *The Pleasure Prescription,* the beautifully designed *Write Your Own Pleasure Prescription* is full of ideas for bringing the spirit of *aloha*—the ability to fully connect with oneself and others—to everyday life, whether in Polynesia or Pittsburgh.

224 pages ... Paperback ... $12.95

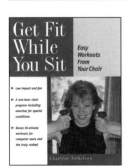

GET FIT WHILE YOU SIT: Easy Workouts from Your Chair *by Charlene Torkelson*

Here is a total body workout that can be done right from your chair, anywhere. It is perfect for office workers, travelers, and those with age-related movement limitations or special conditions. The book offers three programs. *The One-Hour Chair Program* is a full-body, low-impact workout that includes light aerobics and exercises to be done with or without weights. The *5-Day Short Program* features five compact workouts for those short on time. Finally, the *Ten-Minute Miracles* is a group of easy-to-do exercises perfect for anyone on the go.

160 pages ... 212 b/w photos ... Paperback $12.95 ... Hard Cover $22.95

***To order, or for our FREE catalog of books, please see last page
or call 1-800-266-5592. Prices subject to change.***

ORDER FORM

10%	DISCOUNT on orders of $50 or more —
20%	DISCOUNT on orders of $150 or more —
30%	DISCOUNT on orders of $500 or more —

On cost of books for fully prepaid orders

NAME

ADDRESS

CITY/STATE   ZIP/POSTCODE

PHONE   COUNTRY (outside of U.S.)

TITLE	QTY	PRICE	TOTAL
Joseph H. Pilates' Techniques... (paperback)		@ $19.95	
Joseph H. Pilates' Techniques... (spiral bound)		@ $29.95	

Prices subject to change without notice

Please list other titles below:

		@ $	
		@ $	
		@ $	
		@ $	
		@ $	

Please order all Pilates Institute of Australasia products directly from them, using their order forms.

Shipping Costs:
First book: $3.00 by book post ($4.50 by UPS, Priority Mail, or to ship outside the U.S.)
Each additional book: $1.00
For rush orders and bulk shipments call us at (800) 266-5592

TOTAL	
Less discount @____%	(_____)
TOTAL COST OF BOOKS	
Calif. residents add sales tax	
Shipping & handling	
TOTAL ENCLOSED	

Please pay in U.S. funds only

❑ Check ❑ Money Order ❑ Visa ❑ Mastercard ❑ Discover

Card # _____ Exp. date _____

Signature _____

Complete and mail to:
Hunter House Inc., Publishers
PO Box 2914, Alameda CA 94501-0914
Orders: (800) 266-5592 email: ordering@hunterhouse.com
Phone (510) 865-5282 Fax (510) 865-4295
❑ Check here to receive our FREE book catalog

CPM 7/00